ADVANCE PRAISE FOR TRACI D. MITCHELL AND *THE BELLY BURN PLAN*

"I've known Traci for over ten years, throughout which she's remained passionate about diet and exercise. Traci connects with people who face weight loss challenges by simply and easily breaking down how specific foods behave in the body, particularly as it relates to visceral fat. I'm a believer in an integrative approach in working with my patients, which is why I'm happy to refer them to Traci and her progressive approach to nutrition and fitness. Every patient that has had an opportunity to work with Traci has had a productive and positive experience."

—ABBIE ROTH, MD
NORTHWESTERN MEMORIAL HOSPITAL

"Traci is a hidden gem in the world of diet and exercise. As a contestant on *The Biggest Loser*, and someone who greatly values fitness and nutrition myself, I find Traci's approach and advice both relatable and reliable. I'm confident her contributions in publishing will reach the masses, preaching her style of no-nonsense clean eating and tough (but always worth it) workouts."

—COURTNEY CROZIER
***THE BIGGEST LOSER* SEASON 11**

The Belly Burn Plan

6 WEEKS TO A LEAN, FIT AND HEALTHY BODY

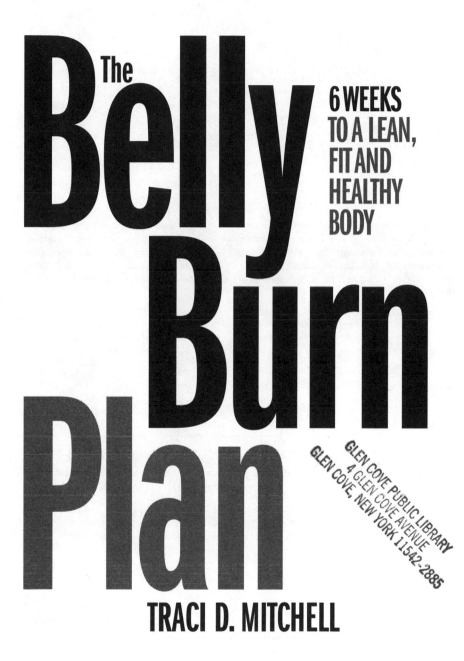

TRACI D. MITCHELL

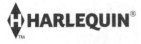

THE BELLY BURN PLAN

ISBN-13: 978-0-373-89323-2

© 2015 by Traci D. Mitchell

Library of Congress Cataloging-in-Publication Data

Mitchell, Traci D.

 The belly burn plan : six weeks to a lean, fit and healthy body / Traci D. Mitchell.

  pages cm

 Includes index.

  Summary: "Personal trainer and weight loss coach Traci D. Mitchell helps readers say good-bye to unsightly and lethal belly fat with an easy-to-follow diet and exercise program rooted in body type-specific eating, high intensity interval training (HIIT), and healthy lifestyle choices"--Provided by publisher.

 ISBN 978-0-373-89323-2 (hardback)

 1. Reducing diets. 2. Reducing diets--Recipes. 3. Reducing exercises. 4. Weight loss. 5. Abdomen. I. Title.

 RM222.2.M546 2015

 613.2'5--dc23

                    2014037922

www.Harlequin.com

This book is dedicated to my amazing grandmothers,
Edna and Darlene—two of the strongest,
yet loving women I've ever known.

Contents

Introduction

Welcome to *The Belly Burn Plan*!

No one gets out of bed in the morning and says, "Today I'm going to eat a bunch of junk that will make me feel horrible, throw off my hormones and add a little extra fat around my belly area. Then after I'm done demolishing my diet, I'm going to sit around all day and do nothing helpful to get my body moving." We just don't think like this. In fact, I'd argue the opposite is true! We're highly motivated to eat right and we want to move more, but millions of us do exactly the opposite, oftentimes without even knowing it.

Misinformation runs rampant about what we should and shouldn't eat. Sometimes the worst food offenders are disguised with labels touted as healthy or good for you. Indeed, most food in your local grocery store isn't actually food at all. It's a combination of different ingredients, frequently made in a lab, mixed together to look, smell and taste a certain way. Food products are *designed* to entice you in hopes you'll buy, eat and come back for more with no pause for your body's well-being in mind.

I'm happy to tell you that you can take control and get your body back on track. *The Belly Burn Plan* will help you lose weight in a controlled and sustained way that will not only have you *looking* better but *feeling* better, too! I'd like you to start with a clean slate, ignoring all the mixed messages you've heard about diets. I'd also like you to put your trust in me when it comes to exercise, another valuable component of *The Belly Burn Plan*. Stop all of your slow cardio workouts and push your body with the interval-style workouts in the pages that follow. In a few short weeks, your body will reap incredible benefits.

Very soon, you'll meet Jenny. She's a mom with a couple of school-age children. She loves her family very much, but most days she's ready to pull her hair out trying to find balance between her daily responsibilities and her own personal needs. She's gained quite a bit of weight in recent years, is often sick and can't seem to find the energy that she once had. Throughout most of the book, you'll follow along with Jenny and the changes she makes in her life to regain her health and lose weight.

Belly fat has the potential to affect anyone—men and women, young and old. Unlike fat stored elsewhere throughout the body, belly fat is by far the most detrimental to our health. Fortunately, there is a lot we can do to manage out-of-control belly fat. Following a healthy diet and exercise plan, while eliminating processed foods, can make a profound impact almost immediately.

The Belly Burn Plan is a Lifestyle

Before you embark on *The Belly Burn Plan*, it's important you understand a couple of things: this program is not a diet and it's not a "lose weight quick" program. You won't starve yourself and you won't work out seven days a week, either. Rather, it's a *lifestyle* that will get you to eat the right foods for your body and exercise in a way that will help you lose weight at a controlled rate.

When you stick with the full six-week program, you can expect to lose what other Belly Burners have already lost, usually anywhere from 10 to 18 pounds. If you don't think that sounds like a lot, I like to tell people to go to the store and pick up a gallon or two of water, then carry them around all day. Two gallons of water weigh about 16 pounds. I don't know about you, but I think hauling around that much extra weight is hard work!

The great thing about *The Belly Burn Plan* is that you'll lose fat, not muscle. Your metabolism will be more efficient and you'll have more energy than you had before starting the program!

The Key to Lasting Weight Loss

A big part of losing weight and keeping it off is understanding *how* your body gained weight in the first place. Processed foods, crazy diets, excessive stress and not getting enough activity are all to blame. Since no two people eat exactly the same, experience the same type of stress, or exercise the same, *The Belly Burn Plan* includes plans based on your individual body type. There are four individual mini-programs developed based on where your body tends to accumulate fat. Coming up you'll read more about the four types: the Apple, the Pear, the Inverted Pyramid and the Hourglass. While each of these body types will follow the same general principles of eating clean, nutritious meals, the macronutrients, or the amount of protein, carbohydrate and fat, will differ slightly.

Clean, Healthy, Simple Recipes

Spending time in the kitchen preparing the recipes from *The Belly Burn Plan* will be one of the most rewarding things you'll do through this program. If you're concerned about time or not having enough kitchen savvy, don't worry! Each of the recipes was developed to be simple, clean and healthy. In fact, many of the ingredients are probably sitting in your pantry right now, and those that aren't are easy enough to find. Prepare to blow your taste buds away as you shrink your waistline.

Integrating Exercise

Over the six weeks of *The Belly Burn Plan* you'll tackle twenty-two body-changing workouts. That's three to four a week—and most importantly, the workouts are short and extremely effective. What would normally take you hours to achieve in the gym can be done *anywhere* in much less time.

Getting Smart About Stress

Eating right and exercising are great, but if your life is full of stress, you're not as healthy as you could be. Stress levels, sleep and time management all play a role in your body's ability to lose unwanted inches. The lifestyle section of *The Belly Burn Plan* gives you the tools you can use to create balance and reduce stress.

The Belly Burn Plan is your roadmap to a healthy, happy body. It's up to you to turn the ignition on and get moving. Let's go!

Part I:
The Belly Burn Plan Principles

"I am so thrilled with the inches off my waist. I went from 45 inches to 38 inches."

"*The Belly Burn Plan* is amazing! The weight fell off, and I didn't feel deprived. I also felt that the plan was sustainable and habit forming, so I am able to continue it. I wasn't bloated; I didn't need to nap; I slept well—all added beneficial surprises."

1

The Making of the Muffin Top:

Belly Fat, Food and Your Hormones

"I was amazed at the results I saw in such a short time with *The Belly Burn Plan*! In six weeks, I lost 17 pounds, and a significant amount of belly fat. My whole life I have been uncomfortable with my tummy, and for the first time I was given food and exercise instruction that specifically targeted this problem area."

—CHRISTINE Z., AGE 41

Fresh from her morning run, Jenny kicked off her running shoes and hopped on the scale, hoping to see a smaller number bounce back at her. Then it appeared: 160 pounds. Her five-foot-four-inch frame still weighed the same as it had a day earlier. Jenny's frustration over her weight nearly brought her to tears. She was thirty-seven years old and more than 20 pounds overweight.

Absolutely deflated, Jenny headed downstairs, tugging at her snug-fitting T-shirt. Her two kids were already dressed and asking for breakfast, and her husband was rushing out to work. She opened the refrigerator for a gallon of skim milk, filled a couple of cereal bowls for the kids and poured herself a cup of coffee—adding a carefully measured ounce of milk. Both kids needed to be at school in thirty minutes, so Jenny just grabbed a container of organic strawberry yogurt for herself. She had a busy day ahead.

After dropping off the kids, Jenny returned home and poured herself a second cup of coffee. She set to work doing the laundry and checking email, noshing on the open box of cereal along the way. A part-time accountant, she focused on finishing a few job-related tasks, and carefully made a turkey sandwich for lunch, with mustard and a little lettuce—no butter or cheese. She popped a cereal bar into her purse before heading to transfer the kids from school to soccer practice, and headed to the grocery store. Always calorie conscious, Jenny filled her cart with lots of fruit, some vegetables, low-fat yogurts, sandwich bread, deli meats, snacks for the kids' lunches, prepackaged egg whites, a package of low-fat cookies, some granola bars and a few staples for dinner.

Back on the sidelines of the field just in time for the game, Jenny felt her stomach rumble and reached into her purse for the cereal bar—a quick fix. She and a friend talked about their frustration with slow, but steady, weight gain. Both in their midthirties, they chalked it up to an inevitable slowing metabolism.

It was after 6:00 p.m. when Jenny and the kids walked into the house again, famished. She filled a big bowl with pretzels to tide them over until dinner. Around that time, her husband walked through the door from work and offered to go to the corner restaurant to grab a pizza and salad for the family. Even though she had just gone to the store, Jenny had no plan for what to make. Pizza and salad sounded like a quick and easy solution, so she jumped at the suggestion.

At the dinner table, Jenny filled her plate with salad first, drizzling fat-free dressing over the top. After she finished her salad, she cautiously ate two slices of pizza, carefully blotting off any excess grease on top. When dinner was over, Jenny cleaned the kitchen and folded laundry while her husband helped the kids with their homework. By the time the kids went to bed at 9:00 p.m., she was exhausted. With a little bit of downtime, Jenny had a glass of wine and a couple of low-fat cookies she had been craving since dinner ended. She watched some TV with her husband, and got ready for bed at 10:30 p.m. Setting her alarm for 5:00 a.m., Jenny put her head to the pillow by 11:00 p.m., ready to do it all over again the next day.

• •

If any part of Jenny's day sounds like yours, you are not alone. Not that long ago my life was filled with harried days of disorganization, eating the wrong foods and not exercising right. And I'm a personal trainer and nutrition educator! I pushed my body to a breaking point until one day I became very sick with an autoimmune infection called necrotizing fasciitis. I thought I was eating right—my kitchen was loaded with "low-fat" this and "diet" that—but I wasn't getting nearly the amount of nutrients my body needed to keep me strong and healthy. I spent countless hours in the gym each and every day, busying myself by monitoring my "fat burning zone," yet never really seeing a big shift in body fat.

It took multiple surgeries and weeks in the hospital for me to realize that maybe I was doing something wrong. I began looking at life through a completely different lens after my illness. Without much hesitation, I tossed out everything that didn't nourish my body and replaced it with foods that helped heal me from the inside out. My workouts changed, too! I was no longer exercising for weight loss; I was exercising to be fit and strong. The result was a healthy, energized body that worked like a fine-tuned machine.

It was my personal experience and the results I saw in clients after sharing the diet and exercise tools I had created that inspired me to create *The Belly Burn Plan*. The pages you're about to read are filled with information that will help your body get rid of toxins, mobilize stagnant fat and live a life that's filled with energy.

Managing work, family and financial responsibilities, and keeping everything balanced, can seem daunting. Oftentimes, the most important responsibility—our health—is left in the dust. Like most people with extra weight to lose, Jenny is concerned and doing what she thinks is right to get healthier. She eats foods that are designated healthy options, tries to control her portions and exercises every day. In fact, this is what most people do when they notice the scale starts nudging upward and clothes start fitting a little too snug. The knee-jerk reaction is to cut back on fat or calories and start firing up the metabolism with added exercise.

So why is it so hard to maintain our weight? Unfortunately, these habits are exactly what are holding us back from maintaining our ideal weight. In fact, the one-two combo of an overly processed diet and too much low-to-moderate exercise is a barrier to weight loss—particularly through the belly area.

Everything you do, including how you sleep, manage stress and eat has a profound and lasting effect on your body via chemical messengers called hormones. Hormones control moods, cravings, body temperature, hair growth, muscle development and even where your body decides to store fat. Controlled by your body's endocrine system, hormones are circulated through the blood, increasing and decreasing levels in response to the way we move, what we eat and how we manage stress.

Today more than two-thirds of the United States' population is overweight. We don't move as much as we should, we eat far too many processed foods and our bodies are forced to cope with illnesses, such as diabetes, autoimmune disorders, inflammation and cancer earlier in life than ever before. By making a few small lifestyle changes, we can take back control of our bodies.

The foods we eat have the ability to make or break our bodies. It's as simple as that. Food can either nourish our bodies, providing energy and protection, or deplete our bodies, denying us precious nutrients and blocking the absorption of minerals. Foods that deplete our bodies are processed and commonly loaded with sugar, refined flours and other ingredients that have no place in our systems. As a result, our bodies revolt, throwing up red flags and sending the troops into attack.

Unfortunately, the battleground is our bodies. In the end, we pay the price by surrendering our health.

A great many foods can keep our bodies healthy. These nourishing foods are unrefined, found in nature and don't come from a box that can sit on a shelf for months without going bad. Healthy foods aren't hard to find, we just have to get in the habit of eating them more often than their processed counterparts. These foods not only help fight disease, but also help to optimize weight, boost energy, improve mood and enhance sleep. The foods we eat have a direct effect on hormones in our bodies. Hormones constantly have their ears to the ground when it comes to what your body is saying. After you go to sleep, your hormones send signals to lower your body temperature and relax your body. When your stomach is empty, your hormones send signals that it's time to eat. When you're in danger, hormones make it possible for you to run to safety faster than you've ever moved before!

Hormones are your friends and exist to help you. They're constantly talking to you, letting you know when it's time to eat, sleep, wake up, throw on a sweater and even smile when you think a happy thought.

In all, there are over fifty hormones flowing through your body at any given time. Hormones increase and decrease throughout your life. In a perfectly healthy body, hormones do a pretty good job sitting in balance with one another.

Hormones are also forgiving. They give you lots of second chances to make up for eating too much sugar, not getting enough sleep, getting too stressed at work and even not getting enough exercise. But when our bodies bear the burden of increased stress, poor diet, sedentary lifestyle and age, sooner or later, hormones reach a point of exhaustion. All the bad habits start to pile up, making it increasingly difficult for hormones to deal with anything.

After years of bad habits, sometimes less, your body's hormones may start to show signs of imbalance. Wrinkles start appearing faster, wounds don't heal as quickly, moods swing from day-to-day and weight starts accumulating through the midsection, all telltale signs of hormone dysfunction. Eventually, more serious conditions may arise, including diabetes, heart disease and even cancer.

All those bad habits you have been meaning to shake for years are not so innocuous after all. Burning the candle at both ends, not exercising right, eating too much unhealthy food and excessive alcohol can have a disastrous effect on your overall health.

In the following chapters, you'll learn how Jenny's life is impacting not just her weight, but her health, too. If you also struggle with weight, a lack of energy and too little sleep, it's not too late to have a good relationship with your hormones again. Happy hormones lead to a happy, healthy body.

Hormones You Need to Know

Of the dozens of hormones in your body, there are seven that you should know and understand. Insulin, cortisol, leptin, grhelin, estrogen, progesterone and human growth hormone all help to maintain a healthy metabolism, greatly impacting energy and body fat. When you gain weight, lose weight, feel unusually cranky, can't sleep or constantly feel hungry throughout the day, it's highly likely that one or more of these hormones are not in balance. It's not really the hormones' fault, though. Actually, it's yours. When hormones are out of balance, something has been done to throw them off-kilter. Perhaps it was a high sugar meal, a few too many cups of coffee, not enough healthy fat, too much or too little activity, or emotional stress.

Let's take a closer look at these important hormones, the work they do in your body, how they are interconnected, and what happens when they are out of balance.

Insulin
How it works
Insulin's job is to ensure that blood sugar makes its way into the cells of your body, giving you a steady and flowing amount of energy throughout the day. After you eat, your liver helps to break down food into glucose, or energy your body can use. Your pancreas produces and releases insulin to help keep that energy moving by sending glucose where it needs to go. For instance, a balanced, unrefined meal will break down into a manageable amount of sugar your body can use for energy.

Insulin comes along, sponges up the sugar and moves it along, getting it to where it is needed.

When it's out of balance

When insulin is out of whack, you'll know very quickly that something isn't right. Shortly after eating something with too much sugar, too much refined or starchy carbohydrates . . . or after eating too much food in general, your pancreas compensates by releasing more insulin than it would have if you ate something healthier or balanced. Under normal circumstances, insulin is released and sugar is removed from your blood. But when you eat a less-than-perfect meal or snack, such as a sugary soda, crackers or a donut, the additional insulin released can cause blood sugar levels to come down too rapidly, causing shakiness, fatigue or even hunger—even though you may have eaten only a short time earlier.

This blood sugar roller coaster is incredibly common among people who start their day off with a low-fat or fat-free breakfast of sugary cereal and skim milk, fruit-flavored yogurt or low-calorie breakfast bars. Those food choices may appear to be a healthy option at face value, but filled with refined carbohydrates and lacking the protein or fat that would otherwise buffer the breakdown of sugar in your body, the only signal your body gets when you consume these choices is to respond by releasing more insulin.

How your body reacts

Short term: As long as you're healthy, your body can handle a few of these insulin jolts that throw your appetite off its game. Consider yourself warned, though. Every time your body releases too much insulin, there is a good chance you're storing fat. The hard truth is all those low-fat foods promising weight loss and a leaner waistline are actually helping fan the flames of weight gain by throwing insulin into a tailspin.

Long term: When you stop listening to your body and continue eating too much food, sugar or carbohydrates, insulin sort of throws up its arms and says, "Okay, have it your way," resulting in a condition called **insulin resistance.** As the extra sugar sits in your blood, more insulin than normal is released to do its job of collection and transportation to the muscle cells. This is when insulin runs into a problem. Insulin knocks on the door of the muscle cell receptors, like it always has. This time, the cell receptors say, "No way! We can't let all of you in. There are too many of you." As a result, insulin turns away with much of the sugar it collected and just sits there. While insulin still works to maintain fairly low levels of the sugar in your blood it *can* control, the cell receptors become resistant to the overall abundance of insulin and much of its passenger sugars.

Insulin resistance doesn't just happen overnight. Usually found in people who eat too many refined carbohydrates or foods with too much sugar, insulin resistance almost always goes hand-in-hand with weight gain. Even though it's fat-free, excessive sugar is devastating on our health *and* our waistlines. It creates a double whammy on how our bodies operate on the inside and look on the outside. But the effects of too much sugar don't stop there.

Eventually, all the extra sugar sitting in your blood accumulates, resulting in **prediabetes,** a condition that is estimated to affect eighty-six million Americans, or 37 percent of the population (1). Prediabetes refers to higher-than-normal sugar levels caused by insulin's inability to clear it out of the blood, but not high enough to yet be considered **type 2 diabetes.** After hitting the pit stops of insulin resistance and prediabetes, the next stop down the road is type 2 diabetes. In type 2 diabetes, the pancreas is unable to keep up with the demand for insulin, and circulating blood sugar levels remain far too high.

People who are insulin resistant, prediabetic or living with type 2 diabetes often have excess visceral (belly) fat due to the excess sugar left in the bloodstream. Additionally, people living with any of these conditions are often affected by inflammation, chronic fatigue and immune system suppression. In fact, type 2 diabetes is most common among overweight or obese people. The extra sugar left in your blood gets stored as fat, typically through the belly area.

Fortunately, there is a lot you can do to reverse insulin resistance, prediabetes and type 2 diabetes. It starts with diet and exercise. If you're someone who can identify with irregular blood sugar levels, or if you have excess belly fat, *The Belly Burn Plan* is here to help. Later in the book, you'll learn how to eat right for your body type as well as exercise at an intensity that will help your body shed fat.

Cortisol
How it works

Insulin and cortisol are closely linked. Secreted from the adrenal glands that sit on top of each of the kidneys, cortisol is normally a helpful hormone. Cortisol helps us get our day started after we step out of bed, reduce inflammation and maintain optimal levels of blood pressure. When your body is healthy, cortisol levels are at their highest levels first thing in the morning when you wake up. As the day carries on, cortisol levels begin to drop. When you hit the sack at night, cortisol levels should be at their lowest point. Think of cortisol as your body's mediator, helping you cope with any sort of stress.

Every time our cortisol levels rise, regardless of the reason, so do our blood sugar levels. When we're faced with a threat, real or perceived, cortisol calls on our livers to release extra glucose (sugar). Our bodies see only one shade of stress, and make no distinction between events that are life threatening, or events that we just have trouble coping with—like that long line at the grocery store. The glucose that is released into our bloodstreams is ready to go to work by providing extra energy for our muscles, should we need to use them in a fight-or-flight situation.

But what happens to all the *extra* blood sugar that was just released? You guessed it! Insulin is released to help bring it back down, and you didn't even have to eat anything to make this hormone go to work. In the case of any form of stress that requires your body to actually use the blood sugar made available, such as running away from someone trying to attack us, well, then, you'll have plenty of immediate energy to get your body moving . . . and fast! But if you experience stress that is the ho-hum variety, like boiling over with frustration when stuck in traffic, then it's highly likely that extra blood sugar will get stored as fat.

The effect of stress on insulin is similar to the effect of too much refined or sugary foods. We can actually stress ourselves into being tired, hungry, overweight or downright sick. When we face chronic stress, whether it's a series of sleepless nights, or dealing with financial difficulty, our bodies can become impaired much in the same way they do when we eat poorly.

When it's out of balance

In today's modern world, our bodies are under a lot of unneeded and constant stress. Financial concerns, ominous news headlines, the never-ending availability of junk food, and thanks to social media, the fear of missing out—all of these create stress that our bodies need to deal with. As the stress starts coming in, cortisol rallies the troops and says, "I got this!" secreting enough to cope with the imminent threat.

How your body reacts

Short-term: Constant high levels of stress wear on your body. Initially, you might feel plenty of energy, to the point where you can't calm down enough to sleep. Remember, cortisol levels should drop at bedtime, but in someone who is too stressed, cortisol stays high, even in the evening hours. You may also find that you're craving more food, or just hungrier in general. All that stress provokes the need for more sugar to circulate through your blood. When blood sugar levels rise, along comes insulin to help bring it back down. When those blood sugar levels finally come down, cravings, especially for sugary foods, kick in. The brownie that didn't even tempt you at lunch suddenly looks like a tall drink of water in the middle of the hot, hot desert. Pretty hard to resist!

Other side effects of chronic stress include increased inflammation, irritability, recurring colds and weight gain. Excessive cortisol can definitely put a damper on nearly all things healthy.

Long-term: When stress is unmanaged and threats keep firing away, the adrenal glands that once did such a great job releasing cortisol when called upon start to sputter out, running low on reserves. As stress remains consistently high for long periods of time, cortisol levels become depleted to the point that they're no longer available. When cortisol leaves the body to fend for itself, fat cells that were once in storage are called to action and relocated to the belly area to help protect our vital organs.

Leptin & Grhelin

How they work

Explaining the hormone leptin without ghrelin, or vice versa, would be like talking about Bert without Ernie. They're equally important, they anchor one another and they don't really work on their own. Leptin and ghrelin play a vital role in our bodies as our satiety managers, letting us know when it's time for our next meal or snack.

Think of leptin as the gatekeeper of hunger. Leptin is stored in our fat tissue and released when we've had enough to eat, signaling to our brains that it's time to put the fork down and step away from the table. In a healthy body, people with more fat tissue have more leptin, and leaner people have less leptin. Yes, you read that right, people who are overweight should have more of the hormone that tells them that they're full, but I'll get to that in just a minute. On the flip side, ghrelin lets us know when we're hungry, sending signals from our guts to our brains that it's time to eat. In a perfect world, when our stomachs are filled just enough, leptin levels rise and ghrelin levels drop.

When they're out of balance

When leptin and ghrelin are out of balance it's usually due to not enough leptin production and too much ghrelin production. This leads to the hunger switch being turned on far more often than it should. The real problem is when the body becomes leptin resistant, meaning the body stops listening when leptin is secreted.

Leptin resistance is most common among overweight and obese people (2), particularly those who have yo-yo dieted or have made junk food a staple in their diet. Higher levels of circulating leptin seem to have very little, if any, effect on hunger or appetite. While no one knows the exact reason why the body tunes out this hunger-controlling hormone, one popular theory suggests that fructose consumption, including fruits and foods containing high fructose corn syrup (HFCS), has the potential to cause leptin resistance (3). This may come as a surprise to a lot of people who start their day off with fruit, eat fruit for snacks or rely on a can or two of soda (laced with HFCS).

Another theory is instead of telling the brain that it's time to stop eating, leptin seems to wander off the beaten path, missing the receptors that would normally signify the end of mealtime (4). Instead, the brain continues to hear "Keep eating!" So we walk back into the kitchen, grab a snack and repeat. This crave-eat-crave cycle makes it increasingly difficult for overweight people to lose weight. As you can imagine, all that extra eating, usually of refined foods, throws off insulin levels, too.

Since unruly leptin is almost exclusively a diet-induced problem, the first thing that should be done is stern diet inventory, removing as much junk as possible. Are you eating too much processed food? Does it contain fructose or high fructose corn syrup? Are you falling into a pattern of yo-yo dieting? If so, you could be making it *more* difficult to lose weight, creating a greater dysfunction of leptin. Later in the book, you'll read about the specific foods that are right for your body type. No junk included!

How your body reacts

Short term: When leptin isn't doing its job and ghrelin keeps on shouting out, "Hey, when can we eat?" weight gain inevitably continues. Remember, out-of-control leptin is usually found in heavier people who already need to lose weight.

Long term: As the body continues to store fat and you continue to overeat, it's no surprise that the typical weight-related health concerns begin to pop up—some quicker than others. Inflammation, insulin resistance or type 2 diabetes, and cardiovascular disease, among others, are all lurking around the corner the longer weight increases.

All this may sound incredibly ominous, but keep in mind; you can take control of your body with what you eat and how you move. *The Belly Burn Plan* provides you with the roadmap.

Estrogen & Progesterone

How they work

Estrogen isn't just one hormone, but rather a group of steroid hormones, including estradiol, estrone and estriol. Taken as a whole, this group is responsible for allowing women to develop feminine attributes, including breast development, menstrual regulation and fat storage, particularly through the hips and thighs. Men also produce estrogen, just as women produce testosterone, but in much smaller amounts than their female counterparts. As women get older, usually starting around the age of thirty-five, sometimes earlier, our estrogen levels begin to drop as our bodies enter the premenopausal phase of life, which can last for years until entering menopause.

Think of progesterone's relationship to estrogen as a yin and yang; they're both needed in different amounts, and play a critical role in balancing many aspects of our bodies' physiology. Estrogen helps to store fat, where progesterone helps to get rid of excess fluid retention; estrogen decreases sex drive, where progesterone increases sex drive; estrogen has a tendency to impair blood sugar levels, where progesterone helps to balance blood sugar levels (5).

Like all hormones, estrogen and progesterone need to stay within optimal levels in order to do their job properly.

When they're out of balance

As estrogen levels drop with age, so do progesterone levels. The problem begins when estrogen levels remain higher than those of progesterone. Higher-than-normal estrogen levels can sometimes be provoked by lifestyle factors. Xenoestrogens, or synthetic forms of estrogen, mimic estrogen in the body (6), creating more circulating estrogen. Xenoestrogens are found in pesticides in food, chemicals in makeup and body care products, food coloring (7), and coffee (8) as well as hormones that are a by-product of conventional meat, poultry and dairy products, to name a few. Today more than ever, with so many processed foods and synthetic personal care products, our exposure to xenoestrogens is quite high. In addition to throwing off our natural estrogen levels, xenoestrogens appear to disrupt leptin function as well—making it harder to stop eating (9)!

Our bodies need a healthy balance of progesterone to estrogen, and as mentioned earlier, it's normal to encounter a fall in both progesterone and estrogen with age. That being said, keeping a balance of appropriate amounts of these two hormones despite their diminishing amounts is a key component not just of our weight, but of our health, too. Progesterone acts like a bouncer at a busy nightclub. It allows only a limited number of "patrons" (a.k.a. estrogen) in at one time. If the bouncer leaves his post, the nightclub becomes too crowded, creating a mob of out-of-control patrons. Estrogen stays in check, thanks to progesterone. But if progesterone levels drop, sending levels of estrogen too high, we're left with estrogen dominance.

How your body reacts

Short term: Any woman who has suffered the throes of PMS by dealing with mood swings, water retention and cramping in the days leading up to her menstrual cycle knows firsthand what it's like to deal with higher-than-normal estrogen levels. With symptoms almost exclusively found in women, when estrogen levels *stay* high in relation to progesterone, initially you might experience ongoing fatigue, memory loss, cold hands or feet, dry skin, water retention and fat retention from the pooch in the belly area down to the hips and thighs.

Long term: Research has shown that estrogen dominance, particularly linked to xenoestrogens, can lead to endometriosis (10), (11), breast cancer (12) and type 2 diabetes (13).

It's important to mention that if you're concerned that your estrogen or progesterone levels may be off, check in with your doctor first. In addition to cleaning up your diet, it's also a good time for you to take stock of the potential xenoestrogens that could be contaminating your body. Ask yourself a few of these questions:

- Am I eating conventionally raised meats and poultry?
- Am I eating conventionally produced dairy products and eggs?
- Am I eating conventionally produced fruits and vegetables?
- Do I eat foods containing artificial food coloring?
- Do I drink coffee (including decaffeinated)?
- Do I eat or drink from plastic containers?
- Do my personal care products (cosmetics, hair care, skin care) contain parabens or phthalates?

If you answered yes to any of these, you're exposing your body to potentially harmful and excessive xenoestrogens—all of which can mimic estrogen in the body.

Human Growth Hormone

How it works

Throughout the early years of our lives, human growth hormone (HGH) is released from the pituitary gland in abundance. In fact, up until the age of twenty, HGH continues to rise, helping us grow, repair and protect our bodies. After the age of twenty, HGH begins a rapid decline.

This is sort of like nature's way of saying, "You're done growing up!" By the age of sixty-five, our bodies produce roughly 75 percent less HGH than they did during our younger years (14). Despite the drop in HGH over time, this hormone still plays a vital role in helping our bodies recover from injury and illness, develop muscle, burn fat and maintain a general sense of well-being. A vast majority of HGH is released when we sleep, and to a lesser extent when we exercise, specifically when we engage in strength training.

When it's out of balance

Even though we can expect our bodies to produce less HGH as we age, sometimes it drops much lower than it should. Our brains' pituitary gland is the HGH factory, normally going into full operation overnight. Tiny workers pour out of the factory trying to repair any damage caused by stress, exercise, injury or a poor diet. If the factory can't open because of lifestyle factors, like not getting enough sleep or not exercising often enough, HGH isn't released in the quantities our bodies need.

How your body reacts

Short term: Since it's normal for HGH to slow in production as we get older, everyone can expect to age, looking a little older as the years tick by with graying hair, a few more wrinkles, and not the same muscular resiliency we once had. Lifestyle factors, poor diet, a lack of exercise and inadequate sleep all influence how much HGH our bodies will produce. If you tend to burn the candle at both ends—favor junk food over healthier food, a sedentary life over exercise and caffeine over a good night of sleep—well, you're probably aging yourself a little faster than you'd like. Initially, the physical effects of lower HGH production might just be a lack of energy, excess body fat, less muscle or even a greater susceptibility to colds.

Long term: When HGH isn't released in appropriate quantities for long periods of time, our bodies start letting us know something is wrong in big ways. Extra fat gets stored through the belly area, wounds take a long time to heal, bone density begins to decrease and stress levels remain high. If all of this sounds repetitive and familiar from what you read about insulin, cortisol, leptin or estrogen . . . you're right.

Even though HGH has its own unique role in the body, many of the symptoms of hormonal imbalance are the same.

Hormone imbalance is not something anyone has to live with. In fact, think of it as a choice—your choice! You decide how you want to eat, how you want to move and how much sleep you get. I'll admit, looking at the big picture, healthy changes can *seem* daunting or over-whelming, but if you approach making those changes step-by-step, it's easy . . . and completely rewarding.

I've had the privilege of working with hundreds of clients who came to me to get healthier through diet and exercise. My proudest moments are when those very same people come back to me a few months after we began working together to tell me that their choles-terol dropped 50 points, they lost 30 pounds, they can see their abs, their sex life is much better or they have more energy than they've had in years. I'm happy to have been their guide, but I assure you, they did all the work—and wouldn't dream of living their life in any other way.

These people aren't hermits who don't have a social life, go out to dinner or enjoy a glass of wine. Nope, they're just like you and me. But they did learn what I had to learn the hard way. Life is fragile and, for the most part, we all need to treat our bodies with the respect they deserve. Food, activity and lifestyle can make or break not just your health, but your happiness, too!

The diet and exercise program in *The Belly Burn Plan* will help you to make the changes that bring hormones in balance, having a trickle-down effect on all parts of your body. We don't have to accept belly fat or an unhealthy body as a norm that happens to us as we get older. Now is your time to do something about it.

2 Get Moving:

Why High Intensity Interval Training Works

"The combination of exercises in *The Belly Burn Plan* has helped me to burn fat, but more importantly has allowed me to increase my overall strength and endurance in running as well as my daily activities. The simplicity of the exercises and the combinations of those exercises make this plan an effective workout that anyone can do."

—TRACEY D., AGE 41

Jenny was committed to making a change. She was running more than ever and had even started wearing a device to calculate the number of calories she burned. She made an effort to work out most days of the week, which usually consisted of throwing on her running shoes and heading out the door for a jog. Some days she ran longer than others. Because Jenny's weight hadn't bounced back to where she was before having kids, she decided to set a new goal. She committed to training for and running a marathon every October. Even though her knees and hips gave her a little bit of trouble, Jenny managed to keep up with her training regime. Her pace wasn't fast, but for the past two years Jenny always managed to cross the finish line.

Weight gain had only become a concern over the past few years, and Jenny fought back by trying to make exercise more of a commitment. She often tried to add in a few extra minutes to her workout just in case she wanted a small dessert later in the day. When she did cardiovascular activity, like running, she always made sure to stay in her "fat-burning zone," and even when she was dead tired or fighting off a cold, she made sure to exercise.

Ironically, despite the fact that she was eating fewer calories and running more than ever, the weight kept coming on slowly but surely. In fact, every year for the past five years, Jenny averaged five pounds of added weight.

· ·

Jenny is a highly motivated woman whose commitment toward fitness should be commended. After all, the hardest thing about exercise is simply getting off your behind and taking action. It seems counterintuitive, then, that Jenny isn't making any progress. In fact, the scale is only going up. Before jumping into how diet affects weight gain, let's look at how the landscape of fitness has changed and how it may actually play a role in preventing weight loss.

Walk into any health club whether in New York City or rural Ohio, and you'll see the most used pieces of equipment are the cardiovascular machines: treadmills, elliptical machines and stair climbers. Most of the people who exercise on these pieces of equipment are doing so at a pace that holds them at a low-to-moderate level of effort. With a few exceptions, rarely do you see people sprinting on a treadmill or push-ing themselves so hard on an elliptical machine that they have to stop to catch their breath after a couple of minutes.

Don't get me wrong . . . moderate cardiovascular activity is a very good thing! Certainly any activity that works your heart and body on a regular basis should be encouraged. However, the expectation that moderate exercise can perform metabolic miracles, helping a person achieve body-shifting weight loss is a misconception.

In 1980, thirteen million Americans belonged to a health club. That's a pretty big number, but it's a stark contrast to the fifty-eight million Americans who belonged to a health club in 2013. The assump-tion, of course, is that an increase in gym memberships would lead to an increase in the number of people with better control of their weight and overall health. No doubt, many do, but consider the fact that over the same period of time, between 1980 and today, the number of obese Americans has more than doubled. And if you're thinking just because they own a gym membership doesn't mean they use it, you're right. We'll get to workouts you can do at home shortly.

The problem is not with exercise alone. People are absolutely eating far too much of the *wrong* foods, and not enough of the *right* foods, something that will be addressed in the next chapter. But when it comes to exercise, moderate-intensity cardiovascular activity has be-come the go-to workout routine, but studies show that it has almost no effect at all on burning belly fat (1)! If you're trying to lose belly fat and have been relying on a forty-five or sixty-minute jaunt on the elliptical or an easy hour-long jog, it's time to stop.

Many people equate the quality of a workout with the number of calories they've burned, regardless of the effort they put into the exer-cise. I once had a client who wore a heart rate monitor to every one of our training sessions. The monitor had a built-in calorie counter, letting him know minute-by-minute how many calories he was burning. Our personal training sessions were largely strength and interval-based. It wasn't unusual for him to burn 550 calories in one hour of our work to-gether. To me, 550 calories is a good chunk of change withdrawn from anybody's bank of energy. To him, however, it wasn't satisfactory. At times, he was frustrated that he didn't burn more calories working with me. After all, he would comfortably burn 800 calories on the elliptical or treadmill moving along at a fairly moderate pace. Initially, his evaluation of my work was almost exclusively based on the amount of calories he burned. I tried to explain to him that the work we did would have a much greater impact on his slightly overweight frame.

It took about three weeks before what I said actually started to sink in. At that three-week mark, I measured his weight and body fat. Somehow in our six or seven training sessions together, he managed to lose 7 pounds and drop his overall body fat by 3 percent. Those results were after only three weeks of training—with no real change to his diet whatsoever. This was no surprise to me. I'd seen the same thing happen dozens of times before with clients.

Today the average woman in America is about five-foot-four-inches and 160 pounds (2). For her frame, a sixty-minute jog at a ten-minute-mile pace (the average American marathon pace) has the potential to burn nearly 775 calories an hour. Sounds pretty appealing, doesn't it? In the mind of the chronic dieter, those calories completely wipe out what was eaten for breakfast and make room for something extra at lunch. If this sounds like a good rationale, there's a problem. Yes, those calories are gone for good, but that woman's body stopped burning calories and fat as soon as the exercise was over. What's more, her body just became more efficient at burning fat.

But wait, you ask, don't you *want* to be more efficient at burning fat? Actually, if you're struggling to lose weight, the answer is no. When your body becomes efficient at burning fat, it doesn't get rid of it as fast. In fact, the more efficient your body is at burning fat, the better your body becomes at hanging on to it. Think of fat-burning efficiency in the same way you do a fluorescent light bulb that's energy efficient; it's very productive and wastes very little energy.

Each and every one of our bodies should be somewhat efficient at burning fat. Fat efficiency is needed for survival. Fat is an essential part of our bodies, protecting our bodies, particularly our internal organs. Within our bodies we have mechanisms in place that force us to hang on to fat. It's when we mess up our metabolism and can't seem to shed excess fat anymore that we run into frustrating difficulty with weight loss.

When we work out for long periods of time—whether it's at a low, moderate or high intensity, our bodies burn fat, that much is true. But the fat-burning benefits of continuous low-to-moderate-intensity exercise end there. When you finish a low-intensity workout, your body stops burning fat shortly thereafter. Long-term steady state cardio has been proven to be fairly ineffective at boosting metabolic rates that reduce stubborn belly fat (3).

The Magic of Muscle

Our muscle, not fat, is where the magic happens when it comes to a thriving metabolism. We all need a certain amount of fat, but muscle helps our bodies in more ways than just lifting weights. Even though we're burning off a little bit of fat when we exercise at low-to-moderate intensities, we're doing very little, if anything, to develop existing muscle fiber, which is needed to turn our bodies into the fat-burning machines that we desire.

You can't grow *new* muscle, but you can develop and enhance what existing muscle you have. I've actually worked with a few clients who were afraid to gain muscle because it would mean they'd gain weight. We've all heard muscle weighs more than fat. That's technically true—but a more muscular person is *leaner*. It's quite possible to have two women standing next to each other who are the same height, weight and build, yet the woman on the right could be three dress sizes smaller than the woman on the left. *How is this possible?* She's leaner. Her body has a greater muscle-to-fat ratio than her friend standing next to her. I'm not talking Arnold Schwarzenegger muscular, I'm talking toned, fit, check-out-my-arms muscular.

Toning your muscles has some huge health benefits:

- **Stronger Bones:** Any form of strength training, whether it's done with body weight, like push-ups, or handheld weights, like bicep curls, helps to give bone density a shot in the arm, making your bones stronger (4).
- **Improved Insulin Sensitivity:** Strengthening your muscle mass, independent of whether or not you actually lose weight,

actually improves insulin sensitivity (5). People with a higher sensitivity to insulin are much less likely to develop insulin resistance, or type 2 diabetes.

- **Greater Mobility:** When we improve the musculature of our bodies, we inherently strengthen ligaments and tendons, too. When muscle, ligaments and tendons are all in good shape, joints are supported, and we simply move better.

You might be wondering, *if my usual cardio workouts aren't burning fat, what will?* The answer involves workouts that push your heart rate up very high for short periods of time, followed by low-intensity rest periods. It's called high intensity interval training (HIIT) and it's one of *the* greatest ways to burn fat all over your body, especially in the belly area.

High intensity interval training has been shown to produce the best results in people who need to lose weight (6). Higher intensity exercise offers you a much, much bigger bang for your buck. When you finish a higher intensity workout, your body continues burning fat for much longer periods of time (7).

Benefits of High Intensity Interval Training

The Belly Burn Plan includes twenty-two workouts, each of which is built around high-intensity intervals. This means you will be pushing your body anywhere from thirty seconds to a few minutes periodically in each of the workouts. The purpose of the short bursts of hard effort, whether they're cardio or strength-based, is to turn up your body's metabolism and get the hormones that help your body burn fat back in working order.

Don't worry! You don't have to be a professional athlete to see results. In fact, some of my greatest client success stories have come from people who have the most weight to lose or haven't exercised regularly in years. By the end of this program, you won't just feel healthy; you will feel strong and fit.

Multi-Level Workouts: You Set the Pace

The Belly Burn Plan workouts come in three different levels, ensuring that no matter what your exercise level was before starting the program, you'll be able to start developing and benefitting from an exercise routine immediately.

- **Beginner**
  You: haven't exercised for three months or more, and may not have gotten off the couch in years. If you do exercise, it's usually just a little bit of cardio every now and then with no strength training.
  How this level works: Every exercise is functional and works to develop the big muscles of the body while supporting joints and ligaments. Don't let the name "beginner" fool you. You'll be challenged and pushed just like everyone else. It's not uncommon for people starting at the beginner level to see the biggest boost in burning fat! Your body is just waiting for you to get moving.

- **Intermediate**
  You: work out a couple of times a week.
  How this level works: The exercises are designed to tone and condition your body, while burning fat.

- **Advanced**
  You: work out most days of the week, and are looking for a challenge that will make a difference in your body.
  How this level works: The highest-intensity workouts in the program are designed to get to those with a strong fitness base into great shape. Slightly longer than the Beginner and Intermediate levels, these workouts can be done in sixty minutes or less.

Get Ready to Feel and See the Difference

The *Belly Burn Plan*'s high-intensity workouts naturally boost your human growth hormone (HGH) (8). Remember, after the age of twenty, your body's production of HGH begins to decline. Next to a good night of sleep, high intensity interval training (HIIT) is the best way to significantly increase this hormone. Every time you boost your body's HGH through The Belly Burn Plan's workouts, you increase your body's collagen production, which renews cells in your skin, bones and teeth. Skin becomes tighter, bones get stronger and teeth are healthy. Think of HIIT as a way of dipping your foot into the fountain of youth.

The greatest benefit in the boost of HGH is in the belly fat department. Higher levels of HGH greatly improve your body's ability to break down belly fat and use it for energy. By the time you have completed this six-week plan, you'll see and feel a difference. Be prepared to tighten your belt a notch or two.

You'll Keep Burning Calories Long After the Workout is Over

When you do high-intensity workouts, your heart rate increases significantly, blood flows faster through your muscles, and your lungs work overtime to replenish oxygen. In fact, you may feel breathless and need to take breaks to catch your breath. This is completely different from doing low- or moderate-intensity workouts where you exercise for much longer periods of time, with quick recoveries. When you bring your breathing back to normal fast, you also stop expending energy fairly quickly, too.

When you perform high intensity interval workouts, your labored breathing leads to something called excess postexercise oxygen consumption (EPOC). High-intensity interval workouts drive up the demand for oxygen in your body, so your energy expenditure stays high hours after the workout ends. That means your body continues burning calories well after your workout ... and you don't even need to move to make it happen.

You'll Have Better Control of Your Hunger

Usually caused by unpredictable blood sugar levels, persistent hunger has a tendency to push us toward foods that are higher in carbohydrates, offering a quick pick-me-up. When you can control your blood sugar levels, you can control your weight better. If you've ever had a problem managing hunger at any point in the day, you'll be happy to know that higher-intensity workouts, like those in *The Belly Burn Plan*, have been shown to improve blood sugar levels (9), (10). When you have control of your blood sugar levels, you won't feel an urgency to eat anything for quick energy, and you'll be able to make smarter choices about food.

With These Workouts, Less Is More

With *The Belly Burn Plan*, your routine of three to four workouts a week is more than enough to get your body toned and shaped quickly. The workouts are more intense, and much more effective, so they require more downtime for rest and recovery. In between workouts, your body will be busy building muscle and burning fat. Plus, none of the workouts exceed sixty minutes. Remember, this is a commitment to your health. By committing to just three or four hours a week, you will begin seeing and feeling the change right away.

You Won't Suffer from Workout Burnout or Boredom

Two of the biggest obstacles someone starting a new fitness program faces are the two they think they'll never fall prey to: burnout and boredom. Have you ever been inside of a health club around the beginning of the year? Gyms are crawling with fresh-faced and enthusiastic people who are 100 percent committed to making *this year* the year they'll whip their bodies back into shape. Within two to three months, most of the gym goers, whom I like to call "sprinters," are long gone. Sprinters have great intentions. They know they need to exercise, so they jump in with both feet.

Everybody wants fast results, but our bodies need a chance to adjust. Ligaments, tendons, muscles and even our lungs need some level of conditioning. Burnout and injuries are a real concern when starting a new exercise program, as they can sideline anyone for long periods of time, from weeks to months. After the momentum of starting the program is lost, it can be a struggle to get it going again.

Another potential hit to motivation is workout boredom—when that five-mile run on the treadmill seems almost unmanageable or the hour on the elliptical feels like an eternity. Even the same group fitness classes that were once so fun can start to lose their appeal over time. Variety is important to any fitness program not just to offset boredom, but to get your body moving in different ways so you're getting the most out of the time you spend exercising and shaping up your *entire* body.

The Belly Burn Plan's workouts are completely different from one another, and the number of workouts per week is safe and manageable for anyone. Changing it up with new and different exercises and varying levels of intensity will keep your mind and body focused on the task at hand.

You Can Do the Workouts Anywhere

None of *The Belly Burn Plan* workouts require bulky pieces of equipment or machines you'd find in a gym. If you have a gym membership and plan on doing most of your workouts there—fantastic! And if you're ever on vacation, away on a business trip or bound to your home, you'll have no problem keeping up with the workouts. Many of the workouts are done with nothing more than your own body, and those that do need equipment can often be done using household items, such as cans, a gallon of water, a chair or a book.

Your body deserves the best, and when it comes to getting healthy and fit, *The Belly Burn Plan* is your guide. It's up to you to take the initiative to push yourself outside your comfort zone to see real change. No *body* is healthier with excess belly fat and your midsection is no exception. The good news is belly fat is relatively easy to move and shed. Big changes for your body start now!

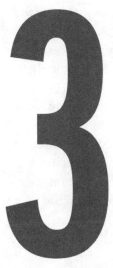

3 Eat Clean, Stay Lean:

Choose the Right Foods

"I have learned so much about food and health since starting this program. I find myself reading the labels and ingredients now and I'm shocked by the junk on the shelves that we all thought was healthy. *The Belly Burn Plan* has opened my eyes!"

—APRIL L., AGE 38

Up until her early thirties, Jenny never had a problem managing her weight. In fact, she could eat just about anything she wanted without worrying about packing on the pounds. Even after the birth of her youngest son, Jenny was able to lose her pregnancy weight fairly quickly. Over the past five years though, the scale started creeping upward. Jenny was constantly trying new foods that offered any glimmer of hope that she might lose a few pounds.

Recently, with her two kids at her side, Jenny was shopping for clothes at a store near her home. Holding dark-colored shirts and dresses against her body, Jenny based her selections on what she thought would be the most comfortable. One of the store's clerks took notice of Jenny, "Can I help you?" she asked.

"No," Jenny said. "Thanks, I'm just looking."

"Well, let me know if you need anything," the clerk said. "It looks like you've got your hands full."

The comment struck Jenny as odd as her two kids standing nearby were both well-behaved.

"When are you due?" the clerk asked.

Mortified, Jenny's jaw dropped as she glanced over at her kids. Pressing her hand firmly against her stomach, she raised her eyebrows and responded, "I'm not pregnant."

The clerk put her hand to her mouth and apologized. Embarrassed, Jenny put the clothing back and walked out of the store.

Jenny knew she needed to do something about her weight gain. More important than how she looked, Jenny wanted to lose the weight for her health. She tried hard to manage her diet by watching calories and fighting off cravings that would otherwise lead to regretful indulgences.

Most of what Jenny ate was preportioned, lower in fat and, at least according to the package, healthy. Most days, Jenny ate between 1100 and 1250 calories. She resolved to lose weight by tracking everything she ate and exercising more.

. . . .

Jenny's concern for her weight and busy schedule overwhelmed her ability to make clear decisions about what was healthy for her body and what was not. Her daily menu usually varied among low-fat yogurts, egg white omelets, fruit, sandwiches with no cheese or butter, portion-controlled single serving snacks and a modest calorie-controlled dinner with her family. At first glance, what Jenny chose to eat may not seem that bad. She certainly didn't gorge herself by filling up on a huge breakfast or by eating too much for dinner, but in reality, her existing diet had a lot to do with her weight gain.

You Can't Exercise Away a Bad Diet

I can't say enough about the effects of exercise. I've seen the wonders purposeful activity can do for my clients, creating significant physical, physiological *and* mental shifts. We feel better, our bodies operate more smoothly, and we're happier and more relaxed, too. That being said, one thing exercise *can't* do is wipe out the damage of a bad diet—whether it's eating too much of the wrong foods, or not eating enough of the right foods. I've listened to far too many people justify a brownie, an extra serving of pasta or a sugar-loaded energy drink because they felt it was deserved after a workout. More often than not, the only thing those people have done is reload the calories they unloaded during their workout.

The food we put in our mouths controls about 70 percent of how we look and feel. The remaining 30 percent gets divided up between stress management and activity. Of course, this is just an estimation of the variables that control our overall health, but diet is, by far, the most important factor. Exercise is a great way to tone your body, improve bone density and maintain good cardiovascular health, but weight loss starts in the kitchen by making good choices that involve unprocessed foods full of nutrients. The quality, not just quantity, of food you eat will make or break long-lasting health and optimal body weight.

Is a Calorie Just a Calorie?

Far too often, we get caught up in basing the quality of our diet strictly on the number of calories we eat—no matter where the food comes from. Calories are a form of energy that the body can store as fat or use as fuel to help perform different functions, including digestion, energy production and muscular development. The greater the quality of the calorie, the easier it is for your body to do its job.

The common "calories in, calories out" mentality limits our thinking to body weight without much regard for health. Since your health greatly impacts your body weight, this way of thinking has to change. People who eat a diet based on quantity of food versus quality of food often end up unhealthy. They have sluggish digestion, poor energy and more body fat. Needless to say, these bodies are much more prone to gaining weight. So even if you strictly adhere to a diet limited to 1500 calories, if you're not paying much attention to what's actually in your food, you'll have a harder time reaching an optimal weight.

A calorie is not just a calorie: A 200 calorie bowl of salad, for instance, gets used by your body a lot differently than a 200 calorie bowl of corn chips. One is nourishing, providing minerals, nutrients and healthy fats. The other is depleting, leaching nutrients from your body while loading it with preservatives and unhealthy fats. It's so important to choose the right foods. Fortunately, healthy foods are everywhere; you just need to know where to look. You may have to play ingredient detective for the first few shopping trips until you're able to separate the good from the bad. Let's do some investigating.

Real Food vs. Food Products

When it comes to choosing the right foods, you as a consumer face an uphill battle put in place by food companies that want to persuade you to buy their products at all costs. In fact, some of the healthiest *sounding* foods on the market today are full of ingredients that are actually toxic to your body. Figuring out what to avoid and what to eat starts with getting to know your food.

There is a big difference between real food and food products. Real food is usually a single ingredient food, like a potato. A potato is just a potato until it's sliced thin, deep-fried, fan-dried and loaded with lots of salt, chemical flavor enhancers and preservatives. In the blink of an eye, the nutritional value of the potato is lost. Enter the potato chip, a much less healthy descendent of the potato, and a junk food that we all know is not good for us.

Unfortunately, there isn't much of a difference between those unhealthy potato chips and most of the preserved foods on grocery store shelves—regardless of how many "healthy" keywords are featured on the label. Sure, there may be varying levels of fat, carbohydrate and protein, but if you take the time to read ingredients labels, you'll see there is no great distinction between what we think of as healthy and what we know to be unhealthy.

Compare Kellogg's Nutri-Grain Fruit Crunch Strawberry Parfait Granola Bars (1) and a serving of a generic store brand of mint chocolate chip ice cream (2). By including the words *grain* and *fruit* in the name of the product, we're led to believe the granola bars are good for us. The mint chocolate chip ice cream, albeit tasty, is universally regarded as a treat, a dessert or something we should eat only once in a while. With that in mind, here is a side-by-side serving comparison. You be the judge of what's healthier.

	Nutri-Grain Fruit Crunch Strawberry Parfait Granola Bar	President's Choice Mint Chocolate Chip Ice Cream
Calories	180	160
Fat	7g	8g
Sugar	15g	15g
Protein	3g	2g
# of Ingredients	14	13

Not mirror images of one another, but pretty close. Were you surprised to see that the Nutri-Grain bar has the same amount of sugar as a serving of ice cream? It might also surprise you to know that one of the ingredients in the Nutri-Grain bar is trans fats (listed as partially hydrogenated palm kernel and palm oil), arguably one of the most dangerous ingredients out there, and prevalent in many processed foods today.

This label comparison does not mean you should swap granola bars for mint chocolate chip ice cream. The takeaway here is that both have a fair share of processed ingredients, not to mention plenty of sugar. But it's important to look beyond the labels and buy things based on quality of ingredients.

Nutri-Grain Fruit Crunch Strawberry Parfait Granola Bar Ingredients:

WHOLE GRAIN OATS, SUGAR, VEGETABLE OIL (PALM, PARTIALLY HYDROGENATED PALM KERNEL AND PALM OIL WITH TBHQ FOR FRESHNESS), SWEETENED DRIED CRANBERRIES (CRANBERRIES, SUGAR, GLYCERINE, SUNFLOWER OIL), HONEY, CONTAINS 2% OR LESS OF NATURAL AND ARTIFICIAL FLAVORS, CALCIUM CARBONATE, NONFAT YOGURT POWDER (CULTURED NONFAT MILK [HEAT-TREATED AFTER CULTURING]), SALT, NONFAT MILK, STRAWBERRY PUREE CONCENTRATE, SOY LECITHIN, WHEY, BAKING SODA, PEANUT FLOUR.

President's Choice Mint Chocolate Chip Ice Cream Ingredients:

CREAM, MILK, SUGAR, CHOCOLATE PIECES (SUGAR, UNSWEETENED CHOCOLATE, COCOA BUTTER, SOY LECITHIN, VANILLA EXTRACT, SALT), MODIFIED MILK INGREDIENTS, GLUCOSE SOLIDS, SOY MONO- AND DIGLYCERIDES, CELLULOSE GUM, GUAR GUM, POLYSORBATE 80, CARRAGEENAN, NATURAL FLAVOUR, SODIUM COPPER CLOROPHYLLIN.

I already mentioned the trans fats, but the granola bars are also full of artificial sweeteners. The ice cream, on the other hand, is equally heavy on sugar.

It's easy to be misled by labels on food products that are marketed under the false veil of health. Packaging with words and phrases like *healthy, low-fat, whole grains, high fiber,* and of course, *natural* makes us feel good about our purchase and hopeful about our diet. The same goes for *organic.* Boil organic foods down to packages that sit on store shelves for long periods of time and the result is a product that may be healthier than its conventionally produced counterpart, but still isn't the best choice when it comes to what our bodies need.

The Two Ingredients Most Responsible for Our Bulging Waistlines

There is very little debate that we eat a lot of grains and sugar in the United States. A little later in this chapter I'll get to how grains, particularly refined grains and sugar, play a role in inflammation, making it much more difficult, if not impossible, for even the most conscientious person to shed unwanted pounds. But first, just how much grain and sugar are we eating?

The grain industry went through a tremendous growth period between 1950 and 2000 with annual grain consumption increasing from 155 pounds per person to 200 pounds per person (3). A vast majority of the grains consumed is wheat. In fact, the average American eats 132.5 pounds of wheat every year (4). That's a lot—especially considering much of what's eaten is refined.

If the amount of grains consumed per person has your head spinning, then hold on tight, because we eat even more sugar. Every year the average American eats about 152 pounds of sugar (3), or about 3 pounds a week. The American Heart Association recommends that children consume no more than three teaspoons of sugar a day, women consume no more than six and men consume no more than nine (5). Despite our willingness to spend more on healthier-sounding foods, the average American is consuming far more sugar than our bodies can handle. Approximately forty-two teaspoons of sugar make it down the hatch each and every day!

You may be wondering where these massive amounts of grains and sugar come from. Let's take a look at common sources of these ingredients.

Refined Grains

Culprit Foods: Pasta, bread, crackers, cereal, wraps, white rice and many snack foods.

How Your Body Responds: Foods that are high in refined grains are higher on the glycemic index and get converted to sugar much quicker in your body. This creates a spike in your body's insulin levels, leading to unruly cravings, low energy and more eating. Refined grains give your body a big shot of refined carbohydrates, which turn into sugar that we just don't need. If your body doesn't use this extra sugar we gain weight, and that extra weight is usually stored as fat.

Refined grains have also been stripped of many nutrients that would otherwise be found in their whole grain counterparts. Fiber, iron and B vitamins are a few essential nutrients that are removed on the food assembly line en route to the package you see on the shelf. Don't be fooled by the word *enriched*, or the small amounts of the same nutrients that have been pumped back into the product at the end of processing. It's nowhere near the amount of nutrition you actually need— and would receive—from a real food versus a food product.

Watch Out For: Common refined grain offenders. Labels with the words *whole grain* or *whole wheat* do not guarantee that the food inside is unrefined. Keep an eye out for these foods that can still send your blood sugar levels on an undesirable roller coaster ride:

- Cookies, Cakes and Pastries
- Enriched Breads, Rolls & Wraps
- Instant Oatmeal
- Instant Rice
- Pasta
- Tortillas

Seek Out Clean, Unrefined Options: These foods are not refined and therefore break down more slowly than their refined counterparts, which helps to give your body sustained energy it can use. A few of my favorites include:

- Old-Fashioned Oatmeal
- Quinoa
- Wild Rice
- Millet
- Buckwheat

Sugar

Culprit Foods: Bread, salad dressing, yogurt, sports drinks, low-calorie single-serving snack packs, cereal, fruit snacks, juice and smoothies.
How Your Body Responds: Similar to the refined grains that throw off your body's blood sugar levels, sugar—in any form—wreaks the same havoc on your system. What's more, sugar is extremely addictive (6), which makes it challenging to cut back on these foods, much less elimi-

nate them entirely. People who consume diets that are high in sugar are at greater risk of developing heart disease (7), elevated triglycerides (8) and obesity (9) . . . even if the foods commonly eaten are very low in fat. **Watch Out For:** Sugar by another name. Our bodies still treat sugar like sugar, whether it's organic or conventional. If you're trying to eat lower in sugar and the food you're looking at contains one of these ingredients, put it back:

- Barley Malt Syrup
- Beet Sugar
- Brown Rice Sugar
- Corn Syrup
- Dextrose
- Evaporated Cane Juice
- Fructose
- Fruit Juice Concentrate
- Glucose
- High Fructose Corn Syrup
- Honey
- Lactose
- Maltose
- Molasses
- Sorghum Syrup
- Sucrose

Seek Out Healthy Options: You want something sweet, so what can you eat? That's the million-dollar question. The more sugar we eat, the less sensitive we are to its taste, so even foods that are naturally sweet, such as fruits, don't have as much of a kick unless they're laced with added sugar. Think this sounds unnatural? It is, but it's something we've become accustomed to. Just look at the amount of fruit-flavored yogurt, fruit snacks or sugar-enhanced teas and coffee drinks we consume.

Natural, *unrefined* sugars are always going to be the smartest option. But it's a good idea to cut back on your overall sugar consumption so you can taste the difference. One of the first things my *Belly Burn* clients tell me after they complete the program is how much *less* sugar they actually need to eat to taste the sweetness. They've kicked their addiction!

If you really have a hankering for something sweet, try to make it as clean as possible. Here are a few suggestions:

- Dark Chocolate (at least 70 percent cocoa)
- Fresh Fruit
- Agave Nectar (just a little)

Fruit can be healthy, but its main sugar is called fructose, which is closely tied to obesity (9), insulin resistance and high triglycerides (8), increasing your risk of heart disease (7) even if eaten in moderate amounts. If you're facing metabolic concerns and having a tough time getting your waistline under control, cutting back on fruit for the time being might be just what your body needs. More on this in Chapters 4 and 5.

The Facts About Fat

Nearly everyone who is trying to lose weight today has been indoctrinated to believe that eating a low-fat diet is not only good for you, but downright healthy! The number of egg yolks that have gone to waste in the name of health is shameful. One of the main reasons people try to cut back on fat is because they think it *creates* fat. Thankfully, that's not how the human body works. Dietary fat is not the same as any form of our body fat, not even a little bit. Nonetheless, millions of people go out of their way to avoid this all-important macronutrient. Not only does fat help us better manage our appetite and control cravings, but it also makes it possible to absorb many minerals and nutrients, including vitamins A, D, E and K. Fat also helps our bodies to regulate hormones and energy production.

The amount of fat you should eat is dependent on your body type, which we'll get to in the next chapter. Regardless of your shape, *everyone* should eat a fair share of good-for-you fat.

The Benefits of Unprocessed Fats

When it comes to getting the most from the foods you eat, quality counts—and fats are no exception. In fact, fats found in food sit along a spectrum that ranges from downright unhealthy to incredibly healthy. For the past sixty years we've been taught that if we're going to eat fat, it should be either poly or monounsaturated fat. Because they're unsaturated, we've been told they help to prevent heart disease, stroke, cancer and a lengthy laundry list of other complications. On the flip side, we've been told to avoid or significantly cut back on unsaturated fat's evil twin, saturated fat . . . or so we thought.

In recent years, new research has turned that logic on its head. Saturated fats provide our bodies with much more protection than we once believed. What's more, everything we've been told about eating many types of unsaturated fat is entirely true. Just like refined carbohydrates that have gone through the ringer of over-processing, making them less healthy, refined fats, specifically commercial varieties of vegetable oils, are subjected to the same type of refinement. Refined vegetable oils can be a hazard to our health, more so today than ever before.

Added to thousands of common packaged foods from salad dressings to frozen entrées, fats such as corn, canola or soybean oil are refined and produced into the clear liquid you see sitting on the store shelf. They went through a multi-step process of extracting, heating, bleaching, deodorizing—and that's not even the half of it. In our bodies, the problem comes down to the type of oil that's being processed. Polyunsaturated fats are particularly sensitive to heat, air and light—all three of which affect the oil in the refinement process. The result of being exposed to these sensitivities is **oxidation.** When an oil oxidizes, it releases free radicals when it is consumed. When we consume these oxidized oils, inflammation (10) in our bodies grows, potentially increasing the risk of cardiovascular disease, arthritis, asthma, cancer, diabetes and numerous other inflammatory-related conditions.

It's important to understand the role these types of fat play in our overall health. You know the way rust can damage a car? Think of oils doing the same thing to our bodies. Eating foods that increase inflammation gradually rusts our bodies on the inside and out. The good news is that there are still plenty of healthy poly and monounsaturated fats; the only difference is they haven't been refined to quite the same extent and their benefits are well intact. Eating clean, unprocessed foods is a surefire way of avoiding this type of exposure to oxidative oils.

Unhealthy Fats

- **Trans Fats:** This type of fat is usually concocted in a factory, and very rarely occurs in nature. Trans fats are a hydrogenated fat. Hydrogen is added to a vegetable oil to make it solid and shelf stable. The process of adding hydrogen to the oil changes the chemical structure of the fat. It's now widely understood

that eating even small amounts of this chemically altered fat increases LDL (bad) cholesterol and harms our heart. It's important to note that trans fats don't legally need to be identified on the nutrition facts of the package if they're at or below 0.5 grams. This may not sound like a lot, but there is no safe amount. Read your ingredients. If you see anything that starts with the words *partially hydrogenated*, put it back!
Commonly found in: snack bars, crackers, cookies and frozen meals.

- **Processed Polyunsaturated Fats:** These are the fats that I mentioned earlier: corn, canola and soybean oils. Not only are these three oils highly refined, but they're produced from three of the largest genetically modified crops in the United States. If the fats in your diet consist of this type of fat, it's time to curb it. Be on the lookout: ingredients on food packages are listed in order of quantity. It's always a good idea to avoid this type of processed fat entirely, but at least try to make sure it's not listed as one of the top five ingredients.
  Commonly found in: corn oil, canola oil, soybean oil, nearly all packaged foods.

Healthy Fats

- **Saturated Fats:** The most stable of all fats, hence the word saturated, this group is the least likely to oxidize, or break down, in our bodies. The stability of this group of fats helps to prevent inflammation and disease. Saturated fats are needed by our brains and give structure to our bodies' cells. Our brains are made up of an abundance of fat, mostly saturated. A diet that contains healthy amounts of saturated fats helps the brain, among other organs, to thrive and maintain its integrity (11), (12).
  Healthy sources of saturated fats include: eggs, coconut oil, palm oil, lean meat and dairy products.

- **Monounsaturated Fats:** Slightly less stable than saturated fats, but commonly eaten in fresh or expeller-pressed forms, this group also helps to provide structure to our bodies' cells. Consumption is also closely tied to a reduction in certain forms of cancer and heart disease (13).

Healthy sources of monounsaturated fats include: avocados, nuts, seeds and olive oil.

- *Unprocessed Polyunsaturated Fats:* Some unrefined forms of polyunsaturated fats are absolutely essential to our bodies' health. Omega-3s are considered an *essential* fatty acid, meaning that our bodies can't produce them, so we have to get them from our diet. Omega-3 fatty acids help to reduce inflammation and are associated with a lower risk of heart disease and stroke. They should be eaten regularly.

  Healthy sources of omega-3 fatty acids include: salmon, walnuts, chia seeds, flax seeds, flax seed oil and fish oil.

Whole, Clean Foods

Our bodies want whole, clean foods. What does that really mean? Foods that don't contain countless unpronounceable ingredients and haven't gone through thirty steps just to make it to the grocery store before heading home with us. It's a lot easier for our bodies to do good things with foods that make it to our plate in as close to their natural form as possible. *The Belly Burn Plan* is loaded with dozens of recipes, meal suggestions and even shopping lists to help get you on the right track so you'll know exactly how to eat healthfully. Don't be surprised if you notice more than a shift around your waistline or the number on the scale. *Belly Burn Plan* veterans have improved energy, better control of their blood sugar levels, greater muscle tone, brighter skin and a happier disposition.

The Inflammation Connection

One of the biggest culprits of stubborn belly fat is chronic inflammation. I'm not talking about acute inflammation such as a sunburn or paper cut, rather ongoing inflammation that flares up and sticks around for long periods of time.

Chronic inflammation plays a critical role in weight loss. In fact, if you have chronic inflammation, it will be very difficult for you to lose weight at all. Chronic inflammation can affect anyone at any age. This type of inflammation isn't just arthritis or achy joints; it's also eczema, psoriasis, celiac disease, lupus, Crohn's and even allergies. In fact, when we're overweight, our fat cells can actually produce inflammatory molecules.

Weight gain and inflammation can become a vicious cycle. One of the best ways to stop the cycle is to cut out foods from our diets that create inflammation. *The Belly Burn Plan* meals are based around anti-inflammatory foods. A few of the biggest triggers of dietary inflammation include refined carbohydrates, sugar, wheat and refined fats. You won't see many of those in the plan, but you will see an abundance of healthy and delicious whole foods that your body will love and thrive on.

The connection between the foods we eat and inflammation should not be overlooked. As you might have guessed, inflammatory foods produce inflammation in our bodies. Compound this with a stressful lifestyle and excess body weight, and you've got a recipe for disaster.

Chronic inflammation doesn't necessarily hit you like a freight train. Rather, it can be subtle, ongoing and low-grade. It's estimated that 75 percent of Americans of all ages deal with chronic inflammation on a daily basis. If you have any of the following conditions, you've got chronic inflammation:

- Allergies
- Asthma
- Eczema
- Excess Weight (yes, being overweight is being inflamed)

- Heart Disease
- Lupus
- Psoriasis
- Rheumatoid Arthritis
- Ulcers

One of the simplest ways to help prevent inflammation is by cutting out inflammatory foods and replacing them with anti-inflammatory foods.

It's important to note that just because a food is anti-inflammatory does not mean you won't react to it. Many people are sensitive to certain foods that create an inflammatory response, such as headaches, bloating, water retention, nasal congestion, fatigue, etc. Do your best to eat largely anti-inflammatory, but pay attention to how your body reacts to what you eat as well. If you suspect you might be sensitive to a specific food, try to eliminate it for several days. Afterward, reintroduce it. If you notice the same symptoms come back, consider eliminating it permanently.

Foods that are common triggers for food sensitivities include:

- Alcohol
- Corn
- Dairy
- Eggs
- Gluten (wheat, barley, rye, and by cross-contamination, oats)
- Soy
- Yeast (including fermented foods)

All foods have the ability to reduce or increase inflammation. Below is a list of foods categorized by three inflammatory groups: Anti-inflammatory Foods, or foods that fight inflammation in the body; Low Inflammatory Foods, or foods that produce minimal inflammation; High Inflammatory Foods, or foods that have the potential to produce great amounts of inflammation in the body.

Anti-Inflammatory Foods		
Vegetables		
Garlic	Brussels sprout	Olive
Onion	Kale	Asparagus
Cabbage	Cauliflower	Celery
Carrot	Spinach	Mushroom (portabello)
Leafy Greens	Sweet potato	Bell pepper
Broccoli	Leek	Squash (summer and winter)

Anti-Inflammatory Foods		
Fruits		
Avocado	Cherries (acerola)	Lemon
Blackberries	Pineapple (fresh only)	Lime
Raspberries	Kiwi	Orange
Strawberries		Grapefruit
Meats		
Duck	Turkey (breast only)	Wild game (elk, bison, deer)
Goose	Chicken (breast only)	Pheasant
	Beef (grass-fed only)	
Seafood		
Salmon	Halibut, cod & tilapia	Oysters
Tuna	Shellfish (lobster, crab, shrimp)	Anchovies
Herring		Sardines
Spices		
Turmeric	Oregano	Chili pepper
Ginger	Mint	Cocoa (unsweetened, 70 percent plus)
Curry	Basil	
Nut, Seeds & Oils		
Olive oil	Macadamia nuts	Brazil nuts
Fish oil	Cashews & cashew butter	Chia seeds
Almonds & almond butter	Hazelnuts	Flax seeds (ground) & flax seed oil

Low Inflammatory Foods		
Vegetables		
Artichoke	Mushrooms (oyster, maitake, shiitake)	Tomato (including sauce)
Beet	Parsnip	Potato
Corn	Peas	Eggplant

Low Inflammatory Foods		
Fruits		
Banana	Watermelon	Pomegranate
Prune	Fig	Peach
Cranberries	Apple	Pear
Meats		
Chicken (dark meat)	Eggs	Turkey (dark meat)
	Pork (bacon, chops, ribs)	
Legumes		
Chickpeas (garbanzo beans)	Lentils	Black beans
Kidney beans	Peas	Lima beans
Grains		
Quinoa	Rice (brown)	Buckwheat
	Oats	
Nuts, Seeds, Fats & Oils		
Coconut oil	Butter (grass-fed)	Walnuts
	Cheese	

High Inflammatory Foods		
Fruits		
Currants	Raisins	Banana chips
	Fruit leathers	
Meats		
Fried/breaded meats	Turkey bacon	Cheeseburger
Chicken	Beef	Duck liver
Legumes		
Baked beans	Northern beans	

High Inflammatory Foods		
Grains		
Breads, pastas, pastries (white flour)	Rice (white)	Crackers
	Corn meal/corn flour	
Oils		
Corn oil	Soybean oil	Mayonnaise
Processed/Refined		
Fried food	Pancake/waffle syrup	Fruit-flavored yogurt
Fruit juice & soda	Processed cheese	Cereal (including granola & muesli)
Milk chocolate	Canned soup	Ice cream
Jelly/jam		Snacks (pretzels, chips, crackers)

As you can see, there is a big difference between food products and whole, clean foods. More importantly, the damage from food products full of unhealthy ingredients versus the benefits of whole, clean foods that allow our bodies to thrive is increasingly significant. You're nearly ready to dive into *The Belly Burn Plan* with both feet. By the end of the program, substituting healthier counterparts for the sugar, processed flours and vegetable oils you've gotten used to eating will be second nature. But first, let's move on to learning about your body type and how important it is to choose foods for your type in order to get rid of stubborn belly fat, and to balance your body as a whole.

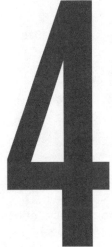

4 Eat Right for Your Body Type:

The Best Foods for Your Metabolism

"I have averaged about one pound a week in weight loss. More than the fact that I lost some stubborn belly fat, I am grateful for all of the information *The Belly Burn Plan* has provided me with to eat a clean diet, and why we should eat certain foods and stay away from others. For me, this definitely is the start to a better way of eating."

—DEBBIE K., AGE 58

Jenny's weight loss efforts seemed to follow a pattern of one step for-
ward and two steps back. A pound or two would come off, but when she
fell off the diet wagon, she would gain the weight back—and then some.
In fact, the longer she dieted, the worse the rebounding weight gain. Still
chalking the added inches up to a slowing metabolism that comes with
age, she begrudgingly bought new jeans that weren't as tight through
her waistline. Her friends, Renee, Sarah and Kelly were struggling with
the same problem—just different body parts. None of them had the same
shape; their weight was distributed very differently.

Renee didn't have kids, but worked with Jenny. The two would get
together outside of work, going for runs and grabbing a glass of wine
whenever they could. Renee always joked that she wished she had Jenny's
legs. Jenny's extra weight was distributed more through her belly; her legs
didn't seem to show any difference. Renee, on the other hand, didn't seem
to have a problem with belly fat at all; most of her weight was in her hips
and thighs.

Jenny's neighbor, Sarah, was a true "muscle mommy." Naturally
athletic, Sarah seemed to be able to develop muscle easily. She loved to
work out, but even though exercise typically consisted of yoga and train-
ing with light weights a few times a week, it looked as if Sarah was at the
gym all the time. In a swimming suit, however, Sarah was self-conscious.
Sarah's physique was much less curvy through her waist and hips than
her friends. When Sarah wasn't careful about what she ate, she noticed
more weight accumulate above her waistline, particularly through her
chest, back and upper arms.

Kelly, an old friend from college, struggled with weight for as long
as Jenny knew her. Frequently referring to her added weight as "baby
fat," the fat was evenly distributed throughout her entire body, especially
apparent in her face. Not a fan of exercise, Kelly tried to manage her
weight mostly through what she ate. Like Jenny, Kelly stocked her kitchen
full of foods with labels that boasted health benefits and the promise of
weight loss.

The four friends would try out different diets together, but no one
diet worked for them all. It seemed as if one person always made more
progress than the rest of the group, depending on what they were eating.
Eventually everyone fell off the wagon and went back to their old habits.

For Jenny, it was low-fat cookies and coffee; for Renee it was nighttime fixes of pretzels and wine; for Sarah it was overindulging on burgers every week; for Kelly it was a daily dose of frozen yogurt or ice cream. Nonetheless, the four friends remained optimistic that they'd find a way of eating that worked for them.

• •

We all know someone who has lost weight following a very low-fat diet. At the same time, we all know a number of people who've tried, failed and actually ended up gaining weight following a severely calorie-restrictive diet. The same can be said for just about every other "lose weight quick" diet on the market. An astounding 80 percent of people struggling with body fat who diet gain back the weight that was lost, and then some (1). If you dieted a lot when you were a teen, you're twice as likely to become overweight than if you didn't follow a string of diets through your early years (2). The lose-gain-lose weight game, otherwise known as yo-yo dieting, is hard on our bodies, creating hormonal imbalance (1), metabolic problems and harmful stress levels (3).

Oftentimes, chronic dieters reach a point where they're so dissatisfied or frustrated with their weight and increased body fat that they resort to tactics that either cut calories far too low or cut out entire macronutrients, with carbohydrates and fat being two of the greatest casualties. In the short term, weight loss may happen—and fast! In fact, the immediate positive reinforcement seen on the scale typically keeps the dieter going for a period of time. But the impracticality of most extreme diets makes the dieter vulnerable to failure. All it takes is the slightest stray from a normal schedule and momentum can be lost. Perhaps the holidays roll around, it's time for a vacation, there was a stressful week at work, or even just the overall inconvenience of eating restrictively force the dieter to lose momentum or give in to cravings.

When we restrict any macronutrient—protein, carbohydrates or fats—for long periods of time, overly restrict calories for too long, or crash diet, our bodies go into survival mode. When we resume eating normally, our bodies store fat much faster. In fact, every time we follow an overly restrictive diet, our bodies' fat cells stand up and do something about it.

Before I go into detail about this interesting relationship, there are a couple of enzymes I want you to know about. Their names are lipolytic and lipogenic, and they're a big part of why yo-yo dieting leads to more weight gain. Lipolytic enzymes help to get fat moving, decreasing the size of fat cells. Lipogenic enzymes do exactly the opposite; they help to store fat and increase the size of fat cells. Typically, women have more lipogenic enzymes than men, part of the reason why women usually have more body fat than men. As unfair as it may seem, men have more lipolytic enzymes than women, part of the reason why men usually have less body fat than women.

Our bodies are incredible machines and always seem to know when we're trying to outsmart them. Crash dieting is no exception. Every time we diet, restricting too many calories, lipogenic enzyme activity doubles. That means our bodies are storing fat at lightning speed, or at least twice as fast as they normally would if we hadn't dieted at all. On the flip side, lipolytic enzymes decrease by as much as 50 percent, slowing our bodies' ability to shed excess weight (4), (5), (6). It's no wonder why people who chronically diet have a tough time losing weight for good. Putting an end to yo-yo dieting is one of the best things you can do to stop fat storage in its tracks.

Fortunately, *The Belly Burn Plan* isn't a diet in the commercial sense. It's just a smarter way of eating that works with our bodies' individual needs, lifestyles and stress levels. All you need to do is follow the program. The rest of the work is already done.

Putting an end to yo-yo dieting is one of the best things you can do to stop fat storage in its tracks.

Hormones and Diet

Not everyone gains weight in the same place. It's quite common for women to gain weight through their hips and thighs or through their belly area, but many others also gain weight through the upper half or throughout their entire body, evenly distributing body fat.

There are a lot of reasons why we gain weight. Eating the wrong foods, a lack of activity, stress and other lifestyle factors are big contributors. *Where* our body actually decides to accumulate fat, however, is determined by something much closer to home. Our hormones, those little chemical messengers that tell our bodies what to do, are the primary decision makers when it comes to weight gain and weight loss.

When we begin to put on excessive body fat that's difficult to manage, no matter where it's stored, our hormones are out of balance. This is why it's so important to eat in a way that balances those very hormones, allowing the weight to come off naturally.

Different foods have different effects on our bodies' hormones. For instance, eating too many refined carbohydrates, such as breads, juices and energy bars, increases our bodies' blood-sugar levels and throws off our insulin. Out-of-control insulin levels are dangerous for many reasons, including their tendency to cause weight gain through the belly area.

On the other hand, too many rich and high-fat foods, including cheesy pizzas, heavy red meats and creamy coffee drinks can lead to increased estrogen and decreased progesterone, forcing the body to store additional fat through the hips and thighs. Even though this type of fat is not as dangerous as belly fat, carrying too much fat on the body puts extra stress on your joints and cardiovascular system.

Visceral Fat

Not all fat is created equal. In fact, your body fat may differ depending on where you accumulate it. The fat you have deep inside your belly is a little different from the fat you can pinch with your fingers right around your belly button. In fact, that fat you can pinch is the same type of fat that's located around your hips, thighs and upper arms, too.

Visceral fat, also known as belly fat, stores itself deep inside your midsection and packs itself tightly in between your vital organs, often creating stress on the liver, kidneys, intestines and heart. Think of visceral fat as an organ that releases its own hormones and proteins. One particular protein, called cytokines, is released from visceral fat in greater amounts. This is a big deal because the more cytokines are secreted, the greater the amount of chronic inflammation our bodies have to manage (7).

Visceral fat also stores and releases free fatty acids (8), which are a form of fat that can either get used for energy or get absorbed by the liver, increasing our LDL (bad) cholesterol levels and triglycerides, potentially clogging arteries. Since your liver already does a great job supplying you with most of the energy you'll need, much of the free fatty acids released from visceral fat alter your cholesterol and triglyceride levels, which can have an effect on blood sugar levels, increasing the risk of diabetes. The message to remember is the more visceral fat we accumulate—*whether we're considered obese or not*—the greater the risk we're at for developing cardiovascular and metabolic disorders.

There are plenty of good reasons to try to get your arms around any existing belly fat you may have. The upside to belly fat is that it's very responsive to the right type of diet and exercise.

Subcutaneous Fat

If you've ever sat down in a chair and felt your flat stomach fold over at the belly button, noticed that the back of your arms jiggle a little longer than they ought to or felt more than a pinch around your hip or thigh area, you're dealing with subcutaneous fat.

Not nearly as dangerous as visceral fat, subcutaneous fat finds a place to call home largely due to genetics, the food we eat and hormones. Everyone has *some* subcutaneous fat. It's needed to help insulate and protect our bodies. This is the same type of fat that a skin-fold fat test picks up. Women typically have much more subcutaneous fat than men, and have a tendency to carry it through their hips and thighs. That's not to say that having excess subcutaneous fat is healthy. Even though visceral fat does the most damage, too much body fat and too little lean muscle mass can inhibit our health as well.

It's estimated that about 90 percent of our bodies' fat is subcutaneous and 10 percent is visceral (9). That being said, visceral fat, that deep belly fat, is problematic in 90 percent of obese people (10). There is a strong connection between excess weight and obesity; those who are over their ideal weight by 30 percent or more are considered obese. However, you don't have to weigh a lot to be concerned. Indeed, it's possible to be "skinny fat," or well within an optimal body weight, but carrying too much body fat. In fact, about 40 percent of people who are not considered obese still have problematic visceral fat and are at an increased risk of insulin resistance, high blood pressure and high cholesterol (7).

Even though subcutaneous fat is less dangerous than visceral fat, it's tougher to move because it's less metabolically active. This can be frustrating, but in the long run, with the right foods, exercise and a healthy lifestyle, the inches related to subcutaneous fat will melt away.

Fat Loss and Your Body

Your body is unlike anyone else's. It's unfair to your body to follow a cookie cutter approach to weight loss, and it's harmful to try to lose weight too quickly. Start paying attention to what's happening with your body *today* and where you're storing fat *now*. What messages and signals are your body sending you? Start listening and you'll get on the fast track to losing sustained weight from the parts of your body that need the most TLC.

What Body Type Are You?

Like Jenny and her friends, your body stores fat differently from other bodies, taking a different shape. There is no one-size-fits-all approach to weight loss. It's time to get to know your body type! As mentioned previously, *The Belly Burn Plan* focuses on making it easy for each of those four types, the Apple, Pear, Inverted Pyramid and Hourglass, to lose weight and feel great.

You'll be amazed at how quickly your body will adapt to your type's eating plan. Energy will improve and weight will come off! In the next chapter you will learn exactly what to eat for your body type.

Apple

This body type tends to carry all or most of its weight through the belly area. The legs and arms of the Apple are generally fairly slender without much extra weight. Even though this body type is at the greatest health risk due to excess visceral fat, the belly fat that's deep inside the midsection, it's easy to get rid of by following *The Belly Burn Plan.*

The Apple Type's common cravings: Starchy foods, like breads and pastas, as well as diet sodas and caffeine.

How the Apple Type responds to a poor diet: Lacks energy and experiences cravings, particularly around midmorning or after lunch.

The hormone to watch out for: Insulin. The key to losing weight for the Apple is getting his or her blood sugar levels under control.

The Apple Type Eating Plan is a higher protein diet. Carbohydrate intake is limited to about 40 percent and the focus is on eating healthy protein and fats.

The Apple Type Eating Plan:
- Is made up of a foundation of clean protein, including chicken, lean beef, pork and fish
- Is supplemented with healthy fats, including eggs, avocado, nuts, seeds, nut butters, coconut oil, olive oil and full-fat cheeses
- Also includes plenty of leafy greens, like spinach, kale and romaine

The Apple Type Eating Plan limits:
- Starchy carbs, to one meal a day
- Fruit, to low glycemic index fruits only

The Apple Type Eating Plan eliminates:
- Coffee or caffeinated beverages as they can throw off cortisol and insulin
- Sugary refined carbohydrates, like sports drinks, store bought energy bars or presweetened low-fat yogurts

All of the foods that are eliminated are known to store fat in our bodies, primarily through the midsection, packing on unhealthy visceral fat.

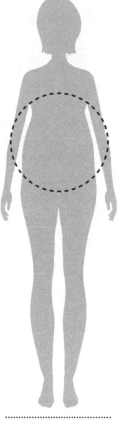

Apple body type

Pear

This body type, exclusive among women, tends to gain weight through the hips and thighs, often with a small lower abdominal "pooch" (this is subcutaneous fat, not to be confused with visceral fat). This body type appears to have a significantly smaller upper body, with little excess weight through the arms and chest.

The Pear may run into a little frustration when it comes to weight loss as the subcutaneous fat through the hips and thighs is difficult to mobilize. In fact, the Pear may notice other parts of her body losing weight before the target area. This body type may experience water retention and suffer from PMS. It's highly likely that this body type is dealing with estrogen dominance. By eating foods that help flush out estrogen while eliminating the foods that mimic estrogen leading to an excessive amount, this body type will lose weight.

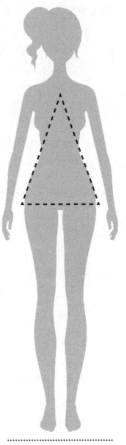

The Pear Type's common cravings: High-fat dairy, like creamy cheeses, lattes and rich desserts.

How the Pear Type responds to a poor diet: While this type may have higher energy levels in comparison to other body types, the Pear will still experience unusual hunger either in between meals or at the end of the evening, after dinner.

The hormone to watch out for: Estrogen. Even though estrogen, as a group of hormones, isn't necessarily bad, an imbalance of too much estrogen to other hormones, particularly progesterone, can promote lower body weight gain. Avoiding xenoestrogens and eating foods that flush out estrogen will help greatly.

The Pear Type Eating Plan is lower in fat and higher in *unrefined* carbohydrates. Fat absolutely needs to be included, but limited to about 20 percent of her daily intake.

Pear body type

The Pear Type Eating Plan:
- Is made up of a foundation of high-fiber vegetables and fruits daily
- Is supplemented with healthy amounts of oats, quinoa, buckwheat and brown rice
- Also includes smaller amounts of lean protein, including chicken breasts, turkey breast and white fish, such as cod, halibut and tilapia
- Incorporates smaller amounts of clean nondairy fats, including coconut oil, eggs, olive oil

The Pear Type Eating Plan eliminates:
- Conventional high-fat dairy including cheeses, creams and sauces
- Conventional vegetables, fruits or meats that contain pesticides or hormones
- Caffeine and alcohol
- Unfermented soy, including tofu and edamame

All of the foods that are eliminated are known to store fat in our bodies, primarily through the hips, thighs and lower abdominal region.

Inverted Pyramid

This body type tends to be shaped like an upside-down pyramid, with broader shoulders that taper down toward the waist and hips. This body type usually carries quite a bit of muscle mass in the upper body, but is also prone to storing extra fat through the chest, back of the arms and above the bra line, in women. Even though this type may not have a defined waist, he or she may put weight on through the belly area as well.

The Inverted Pyramid's common cravings: Salty, fatty and fast foods. This type often craves alcohol as well.

How the Inverted Pyramid responds to a poor diet: This type usually has decent energy during the earlier hours of the day, but then begins to lose steam later in the evening, succumbing to cravings.

The hormone to watch out for: Cortisol. Released through the adrenal glands, found on top of the kidneys. Constantly elevated cortisol levels, released through the adrenal glands, can have a cascading effect on other hormones that perpetuate weight gain, particularly insulin.

The Inverted Pyramid Type Eating Plan is generally lower in red meats and saltier foods, including cheeses and high-fat, overly processed or refined products. Overall this body type eats a moderate amount of protein, carbohydrates and fat, but keeps a close eye on salty foods.

The Inverted Pyramid Type Eating Plan:
- Is made up of a foundation of complex carbohydrates, including oats, brown rice, buckwheat
- Is supplemented with low-fat dairy, including plain yogurt, cottage cheese, kefir
- Also includes plenty of fresh vegetable juices, leafy greens and high fiber fruits, such as berries

The Inverted Pyramid Eating Plan eliminates:
- Heavy meats, like high-fat burgers and dark meat poultry
- Heavy cheeses and salty snacks
- Protein bars and drinks
- Caffeinated beverages

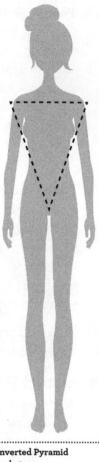

Inverted Pyramid body type

All of the foods that are eliminated are known to stimulate the adrenal glands, potentially producing more cortisol, which can lead to greater weight gain or stall existing weight loss efforts.

Hourglass

This body type typically gains weight evenly throughout his or her body, often most noticeable in the face, but also through the arms, chest, knees and ankles. This body type has a soft, round look.

The Hourglass Type's common cravings: Dairy products, like ice cream and cheeses, as well as refined, sugary carbohydrates, like pastries and candy.

How the Hourglass Type responds to a poor diet: Water retention and congestion. This type may be plagued by allergies and chest colds.
The hormone to watch out for: Master regulator of all hormones, the pituitary gland, which can have an effect on cortisol, insulin and thyroid, among others.

The Hourglass Type Eating Plan is a lower fat diet that is free of dairy and refined carbohydrates.

The Hourglass Type Eating Plan:
- Is made up of a foundation of raw vegetables and fruits, including plenty of salads
- Is supplemented with whole grain cereals, like oatmeal, quinoa and buckwheat
- Also includes a daily serving of lean protein (including eggs, lean chicken or white fish, such as cod, halibut and tilapia)
- Incorporates plenty of spices, including cinnamon, cumin, turmeric and curry

The Hourglass Type Eating Plan limits:
- High-fat meats
- Refined and processed carbohydrates, including crackers, cookies, white rice and pasta

The Hourglass Type Eating Plan eliminates:
- Caffeinated beverages
- Dairy products
- Refined carbohydrates
- Sweets (candy, sorbets, etc.)

All of the foods that are eliminated are known to overstimulate the pituitary gland, which can potentially lead to weight gain that is carried throughout the body.

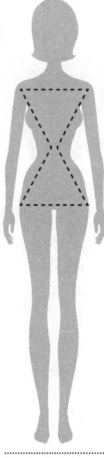

Hourglass body type

Part II:
The Belly Burn Plan

"Just wanted to let you know I hit the 10 pound mark today. I want you to know this is the best eating and exercising plan I have ever been on. I feel great, have a lot of energy and am feeling strong. I love the meals and do not feel deprived of anything. I have even made it through multiple parties without compromising my eating. I have been trying to lose weight for years. I am finally starting to feel like the in-shape person I used to be."

—PEGGY D., AGE 57

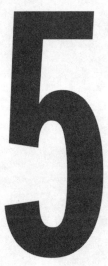

5 Meal Plans

"The meal plans and recipes in *The Belly Burn Plan* are delicious, and so easy for me to follow. Many dishes can be prepared ahead of time and frozen to be eaten at a later date which has made sticking to a clean diet very attainable . . . especially as a busy working mother!"

—LORA P., AGE 41

The plans in this chapter are catered to your body type and aimed at targeting your body's specific trouble spots and reducing overall fat. As the fat melts away, the meals will simultaneously improve your overall health by increasing energy, decreasing inflammation and bringing balance back to your body. Long gone are the days of wondering what to eat. Complete with meal plans, shopping lists, cheat sheets, and sixty-five quick and easy recipes, *The Belly Burn Plan* makes eating clean simple.

Here's a quick recap of each body type (for a detailed description, turn back to pages 50–55):

- **Apple:** Carries excess fat through the belly area, but rarely accumulates any fat through the hips, thighs or upper arms.
- **Pear:** Carries excess fat through the hips and thighs, occasionally in the lower belly area below the navel, but has a defined, narrow waist and tapered upper body.
- **Inverted Pyramid:** Carries excess fat through the upper body, particularly in the arms, upper back and chest. Hips are usually tapered and legs are lean.
- **Hourglass:** Distributes excess fat evenly throughout the entire body with a round, softer appearance.

Are you ready to start eating clean, healthy and in a way that's right for your body type? Let's do it!

The 3-Day Cleanse

Imagine that you're about to go on an exciting road trip. Your bags are packed and you're ready to go. One problem—you forgot to change your oil. You'd probably be able to make it to your destination without the oil change, but your car would run so much more smoothly if you just got one. Think of the 3-Day Cleanse as an oil change for your body.

The purpose of this part of the program is to give your body the kick-start it needs by clearing out toxins that are clogging up pathways in your liver, blood and many other parts of your body. Toxins are roadblocks on your path to success. Wouldn't it be easier just to move them out of the way before you start your journey?

All body types follow the same 3-Day Cleanse before starting on your own customized plan that suits your body type. The purpose of the 3-Day Cleanse is to clear out toxins. Starting on page 62, you'll find a 3-Day Cleanse schedule, including what you should eat, and a shopping list. This is not a fast. It's three days of eating real foods to fill your body with nutrients and rid it of toxins.

Some people experience significant weight loss after doing the 3-Day Cleanse. This is a sign that their body badly needed to offload some toxins and probably reduce some inflammation, too. However, weight loss is different for everyone. If you happen to lose more than 2 pounds, don't be surprised to see a little bit of weight come back on again after the 3-Day Cleanse is over. You're not gaining fat; rather, you're replacing some of the fluid that was lost through the 3-Day Cleanse process. Most people, however, continue seeing a downward trend in weight loss after starting the regular meal plans.

When most people think of losing weight, protein is usually part of the equation. The 3-Day Cleanse is intentionally low in protein and made up of largely *catabolic* foods, including fiber-rich foods that help to eliminate toxins and clear clogged pathways, paving the way for nutrients. This will kick-start your body's fat metabolism, and begin to break down what's built up and release it from your body.

Oftentimes after starting a cleaner eating diet, especially one that avoids excessive caffeine, refined sugar and too many starchy carbs, our bodies can go through some withdrawal symptoms. Because this program starts with a short but effective 3-Day Cleanse, of which the purpose is to draw toxins out quickly, you can expect to feel a little run down. Headaches, fatigue, breakouts and generally not feeling yourself are a few things you might experience for a short period of time. Remember, this is temporary and will pass. If you've ever given up caffeine and experienced a withdrawal headache, you have an idea of what this might feel like. Continuously eating clean and exercising appropriately will not only force a shift on the scale, but also improve your overall health and energy levels.

Just because the 3-Day Cleanse is short, doesn't mean it should be skipped. It's just as important as the meal plans and the workouts; they all work together. If you've had a problem losing stubborn weight, if you have any sort of inflammation, from allergies to arthritis or even chronic colds, or if you are dealing with constant stress, I highly recommend doing the 3-Day Cleanse at the beginning of the program, and then again at the end.

3-Day Cleanse Schedule

Note: Take the time to prepare the Belly Burn Broth (page 211) and Cleanse Dressing (page 215) the day before you begin.

Day 1

Eat as you normally would until dinner. Drink water or herbal tea throughout the day.

Herbal tea recommendations include:

- **Chamomile:** relaxation/digestion
- **Ginger:** digestion/detoxification
- **Lemon Balm:** relaxation/digestion
- **Nettle Leaf:** increased energy/detoxification
- **Echinacea:** anti-inflammatory
- **Mint/Peppermint:** bloating/digestion
- **Dandelion Root:** anti-inflammatory/detoxification

DINNER

Mixed greens salad made with any type of mixed greens and any of the vegetables listed below. Go ahead and make a hearty salad. There is no need to limit yourself when it comes to these types of vegetables.

- Carrots
- Artichokes (fresh or canned in water)
- Onions
- Broccoli
- Cauliflower
- Bell peppers
- Cucumbers
- Celery
- Tomatoes
- Asparagus
- Garlic (raw)

The "add-ons" section that follows gives you additional *options* to add more flavor and enhance your meal with healthy ingredients. Choose *one* add-on only for each salad you prepare.

ADD-ONS

- ¼ avocado
- 2 to 3 tablespoons roasted, unsalted sunflower seeds
- 2 to 3 tablespoons unsalted walnuts
- 2 to 3 tablespoons Belly Burn Cleanse Dressing (page 215)

Days 2 & 3

EARLY MORNING

- Probiotic (see Recommendations, page 284)
- 2 tablespoons apple cider vinegar or lemon juice in 1 to 2 cups room temperature or warm water

BREAKFAST

- 8 ounces room temperature or warm water
- Omega-3 fatty acids (see Recommendations, page 284)
- Cinnamon Berry Smoothie (page 212)

SNACK

- 2 cups Belly Burn Broth (page 211)
- 2 cups fresh veggies (from list on previous page) with 1 to 2 heaping tablespoons Basic Hummus (page 214) (optional)

LUNCH

- 8 ounces room temperature or warm water
- Pomegranate Avocado Smoothie (page 213)

SNACK

- 2 cups Belly Burn Broth (page 211)
- ½ grapefruit (optional)

DINNER (NO LATER THAN 6 P.M.)

- 8 ounces room temperature or warm water
- Mixed greens salad with one add-on

SNACK

- 2 cups Belly Burn Broth (page 211)

3-Day Cleanse Shopping List

It's time to shop for your 3-Day Cleanse. Keep in mind, you may have a few of these items in your pantry, so do a quick check before you head off to the grocery store.

- ❑ 1 bottle olive oil
- ❑ 1 can chickpeas (garbanzo beans)
- ❑ 1 jar tahini (also called sesame paste)
- ❑ 1 bottle unfiltered apple cider vinegar
- ❑ 1 bottle unsweetened lemon juice
- ❑ 1 bottle unsweetened pomegranate juice (see Recommendations, page 284)
- ❑ 1 bunch cilantro
- ❑ 1 bunch kale
- ❑ 1 bunch parsley
- ❑ 1 container sea salt
- ❑ 1 container unsweetened nondairy, nonsoy milk (almond, coconut, hemp)
- ❑ 1 cup shiitake mushrooms
- ❑ 1 cup unsalted walnuts (optional)
- ❑ 1 cup roasted, unsalted sunflower seeds (optional)
- ❑ 1 pound celery
- ❑ 1 cup Brussels sprouts

- ❑ 1 red apple
- ❑ 1 red potato
- ❑ 1 to 2 bags frozen berries (any type)
- ❑ 1 to 2 grapefruits (optional)
- ❑ 1 to 2 pounds carrots
- ❑ 1 yellow onion
- ❑ 2 bulbs garlic
- ❑ 3 avocados
- ❑ 3 beets
- ❑ Vegetables for salad (see list, page 62)
- ❑ Cayenne pepper
- ❑ Cinnamon
- ❑ Ground turmeric
- ❑ Herbal teas (see Recommendations, page 284)
- ❑ Honey
- ❑ Mixed greens (any type)
- ❑ Omega-3 fatty acids (see Recommendations, page 284)
- ❑ Probiotics (see Recommendations, page 284)

Body Type Meal Plans

Your body will be raring to go after completing the 3-Day Cleanse. For the next six weeks you'll find five days of meal suggestions, including breakfast, lunch, dinner and snacks. Of course you'll eat clean the full seven days of each week, but with all the snack and meal ideas presented through each of the five-day meal plans, you'll have plenty of choices to keep you going. You'll also find recipes in Part IV (page 208). The recipes are there to give you variety. While they will be a delicious addition to your daily meals, you don't have to make them all. It's more important to follow the basic principles for *your* body type.

The meal plans are broken down by body type: Apple, Pear, Inverted Pyramid and Hourglass. Follow the plan that best fits your body type (see Chapter 4). Hormones play such a tremendous role in shaping our bodies, and the foods we eat help pave the road for those chemical messengers to follow. Since *your* hormones communicate differently than any other body's, it's important to follow a plan that best describes *your* body type, avoiding the foods that slow progress while eating more of the foods that help you feel great and lose weight.

Good news for those of you giving this a go with a spouse or a friend! Many of the meals you'll be eating are similar, if not the same, as another body type. The most important thing to remember is the foods you should be eating more of and the foods you should be avoiding. For example, the Apple Type Eating Plan will always include more fat, such as a full-fat yogurt for breakfast, whereas nearly all dairy is eliminated from the Hourglass Type Eating Plan. On the flip side, all body types may include a lean ground turkey-based dinner, because it's balanced and suitable for everyone. Apple Types, who thrive on protein, should load up on the turkey; while Pear Types, who thrive on complex carbohydrates, should load up on the vegetables. Once you start eating right for your body type, the weight will come off.

Weight Loss

The most important component of the meal plans that will get results is *consistency*. When you're consistent with your diet and your workouts, you can expect to lose weight (if extra weight loss is needed). After the initial weight loss from the 3-Day Cleanse, it's reasonable to expect a weight loss of 1 to 3 pounds per week of the Plan. If you lose weight slowly, but still lose weight . . . don't stop! If you lose a significant amount at the beginning of the program, don't be surprised if it starts to slow down to a couple of pounds a week. Stay positive and stick with the plan.

Meal Sizes and Macronutrients

Your meal size depends on your size, weight loss goals and activity level. A broad guideline for calories is to stay between 1200 and 2200. I told you it was broad! For the next six weeks, particularly at lunch and dinner, focus on filling your plate with vegetables first, followed by a clean protein and fat. The meal plan will give you some solid suggestions.

As a general rule of thumb for *everyone*, it's a bad idea to eat to capacity. Portion distortion can get the best of all of us. To give you a better idea of what a portion looks like for general foods, use the following chart as a reference:

Food	Portion Approximation
Meat, Poultry or Fish	3 ounces, or the size of a deck of cards
Nut Butters	2 tablespoons or the size of a golf ball
Nuts and Seeds	2 tablespoons or the size of a golf ball
Fruit	1 cup or the size of a baseball
Cheese	3 tablespoons or the size of 3 dominos
Rice, Quinoa, Lentils (whole grains)	½ cup or the size of a tennis ball

Macronutrients, or proteins, carbohydrates and fats, are consumed in different amounts, depending on your body type. They're all important to your success. Here are a few guidelines to eating healthier amounts of each of these three nutrients.

Fats: The fat you eat will not create fat on your body. Don't avoid it. The amount of fat in your diet will depend on your meal plan, but in general will vary between 15 and 30 percent. Fat should be present in every meal, regardless of body type. Coconut oil is a healthy fat we use a lot in the Plan. It helps to increase digestion and has been documented as helping to actually diminish belly fat (1), (2). My top suggestions for healthy fat over the next six weeks include:

- Avocado
- Coconut oil
- Eggs
- Grass fed butter
  (Apple Type only)
- Nuts & seeds
- Olive oil & olives

Proteins: Proteins are the building blocks of muscles. Depending on your meal plan, somewhere between 20 and 30 percent of your calories should come from a clean form of protein. It's important to include protein in every meal. You'll feel fuller longer, have better blood sugar control and greater energy levels. Suggestions for healthy protein sources include:

- Beans, including adzuki, black, black-eyed peas, lima, red and chickpeas
- Cheese (body type-specific, see Chapter 4 for details)
- Chicken breasts or thighs
- Eggs
- Fish
- Lamb (body type-specific, see Chapter 4 for details)
- Lean ground beef (body type-specific, see Chapter 4 for details)
- Lentils, including red, brown, green
- Plain yogurt (body type-specific, see Chapter 4 for details)
- Pork
- Turkey

Carbohydrates: In my opinion, carbohydrates will make or break your diet. They make up the absolute best foods we can eat, but if we're not careful, they can be the worst. Not all carbs are created equal. The right carbs are actually very good for you. Fortunately, we have hundreds of healthy carbs available at our fingertips. Here are just a few:

- Any vegetable, with the exception of white potatoes or processed vegetable products (fries, chips, canned soups, etc.)
- Most fruits, with the exception of very high glycemic fruits (raisins, very ripe bananas) or fruit-based snacks (canned fruits in syrup, fruit leathers, store-bought fruit smoothies)
- Starches, such as quinoa, buckwheat, wild rice, sweet potatoes

Your specific meal plan will go into greater detail about what you should eat and what you should avoid. It will also give you a better idea of just how much fat, protein and carbohydrate you should be eating.

The Importance of Hydration

It's so important that you drink fluids throughout the day. Not only will an adequate amount of water keep your metabolism moving more optimally, but digestion, productivity and energy will improve. Here are some guidelines to help determine how much water you should be drinking every day:

- **Non-Exercise Days:** Half your weight (in pounds) in ounces. For instance, a 150-pound person should drink seventy-five ounces of water.
- **Exercise or High Activity Days:** Half your weight (in pounds) in ounces plus twenty ounces. For instance, a 150-pound person should drink ninety-five ounces of water.

Beverages to Include

- Water*
- Herbal tea (see page 62 for recommendations)
- Fresh vegetable juice, occasionally

Mix up your water with lemon or a splash of unsweetened pomegranate or cherry juice from concentrate. Want something fizzy? Try swapping plain water for sparkling water instead.

Beverages to Avoid

High sugar and caffeinated beverages both have a tendency to throw off our insulin levels. Sugary beverages, such as fruit juice and soda, have a direct impact on our blood sugar levels, thereby affecting the amount of insulin our bodies need to produce. Coffee drinks, black tea (hot or iced) and caffeinated diet sodas impact our bodies by elevating cortisol levels (3), (4). After cortisol levels have been increased via caffeine, blood sugar levels increase and insulin gets released to compensate. It's quite possible to drink no calories at all, from a cup of black coffee, for instance, and still experience weight gain through the midsection due to unruly insulin. If you're scared of quitting cold turkey, swap your coffee or black tea for green tea, which contains some caffeine and is full of an antioxidant called catechins. Catechins in general are extremely health promoting, but specific types have been shown to help boost metabolism (4).

While moderate alcohol consumption may be safe, if you're trying to lose weight, it's best to avoid it altogether. Alcohol stops the metabolism of fat in its tracks (5), giving preferential treatment to the calories in alcohol first. All the calories that you've eaten along with the alcoholic beverages you've consumed will just sit there until they're burned. If you're drinking toward the end of the day and into the evening, there is a good chance that those food-based calories will never get used, turning into fat instead. If you're going to have an alcoholic drink, follow it with a glass of water to help you stay hydrated. You can also try to simply have a tall glass of sparkling water with a slice of lemon, lime or splash of cranberry juice in lieu of the alcoholic drink altogether.

Steer Clear of High Glycemic Foods

All body types need to be aware of high glycemic foods, or high-GI foods, which are carbohydrates that have a greater impact on our blood sugar levels versus their low-GI counterparts. After eating a high-GI food or drink, such as a chocolate chip cookie or glass of orange juice, sugar is released into our blood. Our bodies release insulin to help normalize things, but what often happens, particularly when we eat something that's full of sugar, is that our insulin gives a big push, sensing the flood of sugar. After a larger than normal amount of insulin gets secreted, our blood sugar levels drop—quickly. The result? Hunger and fatigue (6), (7). If you've ever wanted to put your head down on your keyboard an hour after finishing a sandwich, soda and bag of pretzels (all of which are high-GI foods), or if you've ever felt famished less than two hours after eating breakfast, you're probably choosing foods that are high on the glycemic index.

It's important to remember insulin's role in regulating blood sugar levels, but it's also good to consider insulin's alternative role as a "fat storage hormone." Every time you eat foods that contain too much sugar, insulin goes to work, but it also stores fat along the way (8).

Here are a few common high- and low-GI foods to become familiar with. If you have been consuming any of these high-GI foods, consider replacing them with these low-GI options.

High-GI	Low-GI
Raisins, Dried cranberries, Very ripe bananas, Dehydrated fruits	Grapefruit, Cherries, Green apples, Berries
Potatoes	Asparagus, Carrots, Cauliflower, Green beans
Instant oatmeal	Old-fashioned oats
Instant rice	Long-grain slow cooked rice
Bread, Pasta	Lentils, Beans, Quinoa
Pretzels	Air-popped popcorn with coconut oil
Skim or low-fat milk	Coconut or almond milk
Juice, Soda	Sparkling water, Tea

Before You Begin the Plan

- **Start Cutting Back:** If you're hooked on sugar, caffeine, diet soda, alcohol or refined carbohydrates, start easing off little by little. Going from a diet that consists of sugary cereals, coffee, candy and pizza to completely clean would be tough. Make it a little easier on yourself by cutting back a few days before you're prepped and ready to begin. The first few days of cutting out favorite comfort foods are always the toughest, especially if it involves sugar. After that, you'll start to lose your cravings.
- **Remember Why You're Doing This:** I know you want to do this to look great, but secretly *I* want you to do this to maintain healthy lifelong habits and get rid of belly fat, also known as visceral fat, the most dangerous form of fat on our bodies. *The Belly Burn Plan* is a program you can stick with long after you wrap up week six. Between now and the end of the program, your body will be a healthy, fine-tuned machine. Keep your eye on the prize the entire time and go for it.
- **Take Time to Plan:** Planning for this program is the key to success. Before you begin, read through the program and references to get the foods you need. Understand the principles of your specific body type by learning the foods you need to avoid, as well as those you need to eat more of. Prepping your pantry is the first step.

Pantry Staples to Keep On Hand

When your pantry is stocked with these ingredients, you will always have real food on hand that makes for easy, healthy snacks and meals that you can throw together quickly.

For the Refrigerator/Freezer
- *Avocado*
- Berries (fresh or frozen)
- Chicken breasts
- *Eggs*
- Frozen cod, halibut, tilapia, salmon
- *Hummus*

- Lean ground turkey (organic preferred)
- *Plain unsweetened yogurt*
- Unsweetened coconut, almond or hemp milk
- Vegetables (fresh or frozen)

For the Pantry
- Almond flour/meal
- Apple cider vinegar
- Balsamic vinegar
- Canned beans (black beans, cannellini, chickpeas, etc.)
- Canned diced tomatoes
- Canned tuna (light, packed in water)
- Dried lentils (brown, green or yellow)
- Extra virgin or virgin coconut oil
- Garlic
- Gluten-free tamari or soy sauce
- Ground cinnamon
- Honey
- Low-sodium chicken or vegetable stock
- Mustard
- Nut butter (unsweetened, no hydrogenated oils)
- *Nuts (almonds, walnuts, etc.)*
- Olive oil
- *Popcorn (air-popped, organic)*
- Quinoa
- Salt-free canned tomato paste
- Sea salt
- *Seeds (sunflower, pumpkin)*

Italicized words double as healthy snack items, too.

Eat Right for Your Apple Type

It's time to load your plate up with lots of healthy vegetables, plenty of lean meats and lots of belly burning fats. Get started with the following Cheat Sheet.

APPLE TYPE EATING PLAN CHEAT SHEET	
Eat This	**Cut Back or Eliminate This**
Clean Proteins: Chicken, beef, pork, lamb, fish, eggs, white fish, salmon	*Refined Carbs:* Breads, pastas, pastries, crackers, soda, energy drinks (eliminate entirely)
Clean Fats: Coconut oil, butter, nuts, seeds, avocados, olive oil, cheese	*Caffeine:* Coffee, black tea, cola/diet cola (eliminate entirely)
Leafy Greens & Veggies: Spinach, kale, tomatoes, broccoli, cauliflower, etc.	*Fruits:* Any (limit to one serving a day)

Apple Type Eating Plan Basics Shopping List

Here is a basic Apple Type shopping list with just the staples. Add on as you see fit based on the meals or snacks you plan on making throughout the week.

- Avocados
- Berries (fresh and frozen)
- Broccoli
- Brown rice
- Cauliflower
- Coconut oil
- Garlic
- Leafy greens (spinach, romaine, kale)
- Lean ground turkey (organic preferred)
- Mushrooms
- Nut butter
- Nuts (almonds, walnuts, etc.)
- Old-fashioned oatmeal
- Olive oil
- Omega-3 fatty acids (see Recommendations, page 284)
- Onions
- Organic chicken breasts or thighs
- Organic eggs
- Organic full-fat cheeses
- Organic full-fat cottage cheese
- Organic full-fat plain yogurt
- Organic grass-fed red meats
- Probiotics (see Recommendations, page 284)
- Protein powder (see Recommendations, page 284)
- Quinoa
- Salmon*
- Tomatoes
- White fish, such as cod, tilapia or halibut

Even though salmon is a higher-fat fish, it's full of heart-healthy omega-3 fatty acids. Omega-3 fatty acids are something we all need more of.

APPLE TYPE MEAL PLAN: WEEK 1			
Breakfast	**Snack**	**Lunch**	**Dinner**
DAY 1 2 eggs over black beans with tomatoes and onions	Generous handful of almonds or walnuts	Grilled salmon salad with fresh or grilled vegetables	Spaghetti Squash with Turkey Bolognese (page 260), with ½ avocado
DAY 2 ½ cup oatmeal with coconut milk, cinnamon and 2 tablespoons walnuts	Fresh vegetables with 2 tablespoons guacamole	Leftover Spaghetti Squash with Turkey Bolognese with ½ avocado	Black Bean & Quinoa Veggie Burgers (page 247) with ½ avocado
DAY 3 2 eggs over black beans with tomatoes and onions	1 Banana Cinnamon Muffin (page 227) with 1 tablespoon nut butter	Leftover Black Bean & Quinoa Veggie Burgers with ½ avocado	Grilled salmon, ½ sweet potato with coconut oil, broccoli
DAY 4 Whey or vegan-based protein shake (see Recommendations, page 284)	1 cup berries with 1 tablespoon nut butter	Spinach salad with any vegetables, chicken breast, vinegar and oil	Chickpea & Tomato Salad (page 236) with ½ avocado
DAY 5 Green Goddess Smoothie (page 220)	2 cups air-popped popcorn with coconut oil (no salt)	Homemade egg salad made with mustard, side of raw veggies, almonds	Sautéed Lemon and Garlic Kale (page 270) with grilled chicken (thighs or breast)

APPLE TYPE MEAL PLAN: WEEK 2			
Breakfast	**Snack**	**Lunch**	**Dinner**
DAY 1 Cottage cheese with tomatoes over a bed of spinach	Apple with 1 table-spoon nut butter	Turkey burger (no bun), raw veggies, salsa and ½ avocado	Curried Meatballs (page 259) over lentils served with a mixed greens salad
DAY 2 1 Quinoa Protein Power Muffin (page 232) and 1 hard-boiled egg	Fresh vegetables with Basic Hummus (page 214)	Leftover Curried Meatballs with mixed greens salad	Kale, mushroom and onion omelet with a side of quinoa
DAY 3 ½ cup plain full-fat yogurt with cinnamon, berries and 2 table-spoons walnuts	1 Chocolate Coconut Energy Muffin (page 228)	Orange & Green Quinoa (page 274) with diced chicken	Savory Sautéed Spinach (page 271) with salmon
DAY 4 Green Goddess Smoothie (page 220)	2 cups air-popped popcorn with coconut oil (no salt)	Spinach salad with any vegetables, chicken breast, vinegar and oil	Beef burger (no bun), ½ sweet potato, broccoli
DAY 5 2 scrambled eggs with spinach and tomato, cooked in coconut oil	Berries and handful of raw nuts	Leaf lettuce wrap made with leftover beef burger with veggies and unsalted mixed nuts	Orange & Green Quinoa (page 274) with grilled chicken

APPLE TYPE MEAL PLAN: WEEK 3			
Breakfast	**Snack**	**Lunch**	**Dinner**
DAY 1 ½ cup oatmeal with 2 tablespoons unsweetened nut butter and cinnamon	Green apple with 1 tablespoon nut butter	Black Bean & Tomato Salad (page 234), guacamole with veggies	Shredded BBQ Chicken (page 254) and Clean Cole Slaw (page 276)
DAY 2 1 Lemon Chia Seed Muffin (page 229) and 1 hard-boiled egg	Basic Hummus (page 214) with fresh vegetables	Leftover Shredded BBQ Chicken and Clean Cole Slaw	Grilled chicken salad with fresh vegetables plus vinegar and olive oil dressing
DAY 3 2 eggs with kale or spinach, cooked in coconut oil	2 cups air-popped popcorn with coconut oil (no salt)	1 ½ cups plain full-fat yogurt, 1 cup berries, 2 tablespoons walnuts and cinnamon	Lentil Burger (page 250, no bun), sliced avocado, fresh veggies
DAY 4 Avocado Berry Smoothie (page 223)	1 Lemon Chia Seed Muffin (page 229)	Leftover Lentil Burger (no bun) with sliced tomato and avocado	Sweet Potato Turkey Burgers (page 262, no bun), mixed greens salad
DAY 5 1 cup plain full-fat yogurt, berries, cinnamon, 2 tablespoons walnuts	¼ cup pumpkin seeds and a green apple	Leftover Sweet Potato Turkey Burger (no bun), fresh vegetable	Grilled white fish, steamed spinach with olive oil, salt

APPLE TYPE MEAL PLAN: WEEK 4			
Breakfast	**Snack**	**Lunch**	**Dinner**
DAY 1 1 Strawberry Muffin (page 233), 1 hard-boiled egg	Blueberry Spinach Smoothie (page 217)	Quinoa Tabouli (page 239) with avocado	Pot Pie Crumble (page 252) and a mixed greens salad
DAY 2 Overnight Chia Seed Oatmeal (page 226) *note:* prepare the night before	Fresh vegetables with Spicy Black Bean Dip (page 278)	Leftover Pot Pie Crumble	Beef burger (no bun), fresh veggies and sweet potato fries
DAY 3 2 egg spinach & mushroom omelet with diced tomatoes	2 cups air-popped popcorn with coconut oil (no salt)	Leftover beef burger (no bun) with fresh vegetables	Turkey-Stuffed Peppers (page 265)
DAY 4 1 Double Chocolate Protein Muffin (page 230), 1 hard-boiled egg	Apple with 2 tablespoons nut butter	Leftover Turkey-Stuffed Peppers	Grilled chicken salad with vegetable plus vinegar and olive oil dressing
DAY 5 Cinnamon Berry Smoothie (page 212)	1 Double Chocolate Protein Muffin (page 230)	Chopped salad with avocado, egg, tomato, onion, olive oil, vinegar and sea salt	Grilled salmon and sautéed spinach with brown rice

APPLE TYPE MEAL PLAN: WEEK 5			
Breakfast	**Snack**	**Lunch**	**Dinner**
DAY 1 2 scrambled eggs with ¼ avocado and fresh berries	Unsalted mixed nuts and fresh veggies	Citrus Mint Quinoa Salad (page 237) with diced chicken and avocado	Grilled chicken with steamed vegetables tossed in coconut oil
DAY 2 Oatmeal with 2 tablespoons walnuts, coconut milk and cinnamon	Avocado Berry Smoothie (page 223)	Southwest Fajita Salad (page 242)	Leftover grilled chicken with leftover Citrus Mint Quinoa Salad
DAY 3 1 cup plain yogurt with 1 tablespoon chia seeds, berries and cinnamon	Green apple with 2 tablespoons nut butter	Almond & Honey-Crusted Pork Chop (page 245) with roasted vegetables and salad	Leftover Southwest Fajita Salad
DAY 4 Cinnamon Berry Smoothie (page 212)	2 hard-boiled eggs, 1 cup fresh carrots	White fish with coconut oil, lemon, sea salt, broccoli	Leftover Almond & Honey-Crusted Pork Chop
DAY 5 2 hard-boiled eggs, bacon and sliced tomatoes	Spicy Black Bean Dip (page 278) with fresh veggies	Grilled chicken salad with vegetable plus vinegar and olive oil dressing	Black Bean, Corn & Red Pepper Lettuce Wraps (page 246) with ½ avocado

APPLE TYPE MEAL PLAN: WEEK 6			
Breakfast	**Snack**	**Lunch**	**Dinner**
DAY 1 2 scrambled eggs with ¼ avocado and fresh berries	Apple with ½ cup plain low-fat yogurt with cinnamon	Simple Butternut Squash Soup (page 272), fresh vegetables, Basic Hummus (page 214)	Cauliflower Crust Pizza (page 248) with mixed greens salad
DAY 2 Creamy Green Dream Smoothie (page 219)	1 Chocolate Chunk Avocado Cookie (page 282)	Napa & Red Cabbage Salad (page 238)	Chicken Vegetable Curry (page 256) with brown rice or quinoa
DAY 3 Oatmeal with 2 tablespoons walnuts, cinnamon	1 cup berries, 1 tbsp nut butter	Leftover Chicken Vegetable Curry	Leftover Napa & Red Cabbage Salad with grilled chicken
DAY 4 2 hard-boiled eggs, fresh berry salad	2 cups air-popped popcorn with coconut oil (no salt)	Rainbow Kale Salad (page 240) with grilled chicken	Split Pea & Turkey Soup (page 273)
DAY 5 1 Oat & Almond Breakfast Bar (page 225) with 2 tablespoons nut butter and cinnamon	½ cup full-fat yogurt with berries and cinnamon	Leftover Split Pea & Turkey Soup	Roasted Parsnips & Carrots (page 275) with salmon

Eat Right for Your Pear Type

Carbohydrates love you, just not the refined variety. Give your body a boost of fat-burning energy by loading up on vegetables, fruits and other complex carbohydrates, like old-fashioned oats and quinoa. Don't forget to pair with a little bit of lean protein and some fat, too!

PEAR TYPE EATING PLAN CHEAT SHEET	
Eat This	**Cut Back or Eliminate This**
High-fiber Fruits & Veggies: Leafy greens, carrots, broccoli, berries, prunes, etc.	*High-fat Dairy:* Creams, cheeses, ice cream
Complex Carbohydrates: Old-fashioned oats, quinoa, brown rice	*Caffeine:* Coffee, black tea, cola/diet cola (eliminate entirely)
Lean Proteins: A small amount of chicken, white fish, salmon, eggs (whole)	*Estrogen Imitators:* Added hormones, foods with pesticides, unfermented soy products (tofu)
Clean Nondairy Fats: Coconut oil, avocado, olive oil, nuts, seeds	*Refined Carbs:* Breads, pastas, pastries, crackers, soda, energy drinks (eliminate entirely)

Pear Type Eating Plan Basics Shopping List

Here is a basic Pear Type shopping list with just the staples. Add on as you see fit based on the meals or snacks you plan on making throughout the week.

- Apples
- Avocados
- Berries (fresh and frozen)
- Black beans
- Broccoli
- Brown rice
- Brussels sprouts
- Cauliflower
- Chia seeds
- Chickpeas
- Coconut oil
- Garlic
- Leafy greens (spinach, romaine, kale)
- Lean ground turkey (organic preferred)
- Nut butter
- Nuts (almonds, walnuts, etc.)
- Old-fashioned oatmeal
- Olive oil
- Omega-3 fatty acids (see Recommendations, page 284)
- Onions
- Organic chicken breasts
- Organic eggs
- Organic low-fat cottage cheese
- Organic plain low-fat yogurt
- Probiotics (see Recommendations, page 284)
- Protein powder (see Recommendations, page 284)
- Prunes
- Quinoa
- Salmon*
- Tomatoes
- White fish, such as cod, tilapia or halibut

Even though salmon is a higher-fat fish, it's full of heart-healthy omega-3 fatty acids. Omega-3 fatty acids are something we all need more of.

PEAR TYPE MEAL PLAN: WEEK 1			
Breakfast	Snack	Lunch	Dinner
DAY 1 2 hard-boiled eggs and fresh berries	5 prunes plus small handful of almonds	Grilled salmon salad with fresh vegetables	Spaghetti Squash with Turkey Bolognese (page 260)
DAY 2 ½ cup oatmeal with coconut milk, cinnamon and 2 tablespoons walnuts	Fresh vegetables with 2 tablespoons Basic Hummus (page 214)	Leftover Spaghetti Squash with Turkey Bolognese	Black Bean & Quinoa Veggie Burgers (page 247) with fresh veggies
DAY 3 2 hard-boiled eggs and fresh berries	1 Strawberry Muffin (page 233)	Leftover Black Bean & Quinoa Veggie Burgers with fresh veggies	Grilled white fish, ½ sweet potato with coconut oil, broccoli
DAY 4 Whey or vegan-based protein shake (see Recommendations, page 284)	5 prunes plus small handful of almonds	Spinach salad with any vegetables, chicken breast, vinegar and oil	Chickpea & Tomato Salad (page 236)
DAY 5 Avocado Berry Smoothie (page 223)	2 cups air-popped popcorn with coconut oil (no salt)	Homemade egg salad made with mustard, side of raw veggies, almonds	Sautéed Lemon & Garlic Kale (page 270) with grilled chicken breast

PEAR TYPE MEAL PLAN: WEEK 2			
Breakfast	**Snack**	**Lunch**	**Dinner**
DAY 1 ½ cup low-fat cottage cheese with tomatoes over a bed of spinach	Apple with 1 tablespoon nut butter	Turkey burger (no bun), raw veggies, salsa and ½ avocado	Curried Meatballs (page 259) over lentils served with a mixed greens salad
DAY 2 1 Quinoa Protein Power Muffin (page 232) and 1 hard-boiled egg	Fresh vegetables with Basic Hummus (page 214)	Leftover Curried Meatballs with mixed greens salad	Kale, mushroom and onion omelet with a side of quinoa
DAY 3 ½ cup plain low-fat yogurt with cinnamon, berries and 2 tablespoons walnuts	5 prunes plus small handful of almonds	Orange & Green Quinoa (page 274) with diced chicken	Savory Sautéed Spinach (page 271) with salmon
DAY 4 Chia Berry Smoothie (page 218)	2 cups air-popped popcorn with coconut oil (no salt)	Leftover Orange & Green Quinoa with grilled chicken	Turkey burger (no bun), broccoli or cauliflower
DAY 5 2 scrambled eggs with spinach and tomato, cooked in coconut oil	5 prunes plus handful of raw nuts	Leaf lettuce wrap made with leftover burger with veggies	Spinach salad with any vegetables, chicken breast, vinegar and oil

PEAR TYPE MEAL PLAN: WEEK 3

	Breakfast	Snack	Lunch	Dinner
DAY 1	½ cup oatmeal with 2 tablespoons unsweetened nut butter and cinnamon	5 prunes plus small handful of almonds	Black Bean & Tomato Salad (page 234) and guacamole with veggies	Shredded BBQ Chicken (page 254) and Clean Cole Slaw (page 276)
DAY 2	1 Double Chocolate Protein Muffin (page 230) and fresh berries	Basic Hummus (page 214) with fresh vegetables	Leftover Shredded BBQ Chicken and Clean Cole Slaw	Grilled chicken salad with vegetable plus vinegar and olive oil dressing
DAY 3	2 hard-boiled eggs and sliced apple	1 Double Chocolate Protein Muffin (page 230)	Tossed salad with fresh veggies, vinegar and olive oil	Lentil Burger (page 250, no bun), sliced avocado, fresh veggies
DAY 4	Avocado Berry Smoothie (page 223)	5 prunes plus small handful of almonds	Leftover Lentil Burger (no bun) with fresh veggies	Sweet Potato Turkey Burgers (page 262, no bun), mixed greens salad
DAY 5	Vanilla Yogurt Berry Parfait (page 224)	2 cups air-popped popcorn with coconut oil (no salt)	Leftover Sweet Potato Turkey Burger (no bun), fresh vegetable	Grilled white fish, steamed spinach with olive oil, salt, broccoli

PEAR TYPE MEAL PLAN: WEEK 4			
Breakfast	**Snack**	**Lunch**	**Dinner**
DAY 1 1 Strawberry Muffin (page 233), 1 hard-boiled egg	Blueberry Spinach Smoothie (page 217)	Quinoa Tabouli (page 239) with avocado	Pot Pie Crumble (page 252) and a mixed greens salad
DAY 2 Overnight Chia Seed Oatmeal (page 226) *note:* prepare the night before	5 prunes plus handful of almonds	Leftover Pot Pie Crumble	Grilled chicken breast with leftover Quinoa Tabouli
DAY 3 2 egg spinach & mushroom omelet with diced tomatoes	2 cups air-popped popcorn with coconut oil (no salt)	Grilled chicken breast with fresh vegetables	Turkey-Stuffed Peppers (page 265)
DAY 4 1 Double Chocolate Protein Muffin (page 230), 1 hard-boiled egg	5 prunes plus handful of almonds	Chickpea & Tomato Salad (page 236)	Leftover Turkey-Stuffed Peppers
DAY 5 Cinnamon Berry Smoothie (page 212)	Apple with 2 tablespoons nut butter	Chopped salad with egg, tomato, onion, olive oil, vinegar and sea salt	Grilled salmon and sautéed spinach with brown rice

PEAR TYPE MEAL PLAN: WEEK 5			
Breakfast	**Snack**	**Lunch**	**Dinner**
DAY 1 2 scrambled eggs plus fresh berries	5 prunes plus small handful of almonds	Broccoli Jicama Detox Salad (page 235)	Grilled chicken with steamed vegetables tossed in coconut oil
DAY 2 Vanilla Yogurt Berry Parfait (224)	Cinnamon Berry Smoothie (page 212)	Cauliflower Soup (page 268) and mixed green salad with vinegar and oil	Citrus Mint Quinoa Salad (page 237) with leftover Broccoli Jicama Detox Salad
DAY 3 ½ cup old-fashioned oats with cinnamon, berries and 1 tablespoon chia seeds	Green apple with 1 tablespoon nut butter	Leftover Citrus Mint Quinoa Salad with fresh veggies and avocado	Southwest Fajita Salad (page 242)
DAY 4 Chia Berry Smoothie (page 218)	5 prunes plus small handful of almonds	Leftover Southwest Fajita Salad	White fish with coconut oil, lemon, sea salt, broccoli
DAY 5 2 hard-boiled eggs, fresh berries and sliced tomatoes	Basic Hummus (page 214) with fresh veggies	Grilled chicken salad with vegetable plus vinegar and olive oil dressing	Cauliflower Crust Pizza (page 248) with mixed greens salad

PEAR TYPE MEAL PLAN: WEEK 6			
Breakfast	**Snack**	**Lunch**	**Dinner**
DAY 1 2 hard-boiled eggs and fresh berries	Apple with ¼ cup plain low-fat yogurt and cinnamon dip	Simple Butternut Squash Soup (page 272), fresh vegetables, Basic Hummus (page 214)	Grilled chicken breast, ½ cup brown rice and broccoli drizzled with coconut oil
DAY 2 Creamy Green Dream Smoothie (page 219)	1 Chocolate Chunk Avocado Cookie (page 282)	Napa & Red Cabbage Salad (page 238)	Chicken Vegetable Curry (page 256) with brown rice or quinoa
DAY 3 ½ cup old-fashioned oats plus cinnamon and 2 tablespoons walnuts and fresh berries	5 prunes plus handful of almonds	Leftover Chicken Vegetable Curry	Leftover Napa & Red Cabbage Salad with grilled chicken
DAY 4 Omega Berry Smoothie (page 221)	2 No Bake Chocolate Energy Balls (page 281)	Rainbow Kale Salad (page 240)	Split Pea & Turkey Soup (page 273)
DAY 5 1 Oat & Almond Breakfast Bar (page 225) with 1 tablespoon nut butter and cinnamon	5 prunes plus handful of almonds	Leftover Split Pea & Turkey Soup	Leftover Rainbow Kale Salad

Eat Right for Your Inverted Pyramid Type

Ditch the fat-loaded, salt-filled snacks and meals pronto! Replace them with these healthy and delicious options that will energize your body all day long while fighting fat at the same time.

INVERTED PYRAMID TYPE EATING PLAN CHEAT SHEET	
Eat This	**Cut Back or Eliminate This**
Vegetables, Fruits & Fresh Veggie Juices: Kale, carrots, apples, berries, green juices	*High-fat Dairy:* Creams, cheeses, ice cream
Complex Carbohydrates: Old-fashioned oats, quinoa, brown rice	*Heavy Meats:* High-fat red meats, dark meat poultry
Low-fat Dairy: Plain yogurt, cottage cheese, kefir	*Caffeine:* Coffee, black tea, cola/diet cola (eliminate entirely)
Lean Proteins: Turkey & chicken breast, lean cuts of pork, very lean beef, white fish	*Salty Snacks:* Chips, crackers, salted nuts

Inverted Pyramid Type Eating Plan Basics Shopping List

Here is a basic Inverted Pyramid Type shopping list with just the staples. Add on as you see fit based on the meals or snacks you plan on making throughout the week.

- Apples
- Avocados
- Berries (fresh and frozen)
- Broccoli
- Brown rice
- Brussels sprouts
- Cauliflower
- Chia seeds
- Coconut oil
- Garlic
- Leafy greens (spinach, romaine, kale)
- Lean ground turkey (organic preferred)
- Nut butter
- Nuts (almonds, walnuts, etc.) (no salt added)
- Old-fashioned oats
- Olive oil
- Omega-3 fatty acids (see Recommendations, page 284)
- Onions
- Organic chicken breasts
- Organic eggs
- Organic low-fat cottage cheese (low sodium)
- Organic plain low-fat yogurt
- Probiotics (see Recommendations, page 284)
- Protein powder (see Recommendations, page 284)
- Quinoa
- Salmon*
- Tomatoes
- White fish, such as cod, tilapia or halibut

Even though salmon is a higher-fat fish, it's full of heart-healthy omega-3 fatty acids. Omega-3 fatty acids are something we all need more of.

INVERTED PYRAMID TYPE MEAL PLAN: WEEK 1			
Breakfast	**Snack**	**Lunch**	**Dinner**
DAY 1 2 hard-boiled or poached eggs over sautéed spinach	Apple and small handful of almonds	Green Goddess Smoothie (page 220)	Spaghetti Squash with Turkey Bolognese (page 260) with ½ avocado
DAY 2 ½ cup oatmeal with coconut milk, cinnamon and 2 tablespoons walnuts	Fresh vegetables with 2 tablespoons guacamole	Leftover Spaghetti Squash with Turkey Bolognese with ½ avocado	Black Bean & Quinoa Veggie Burger (page 247) with ½ avocado
DAY 3 1 cup low-fat cottage cheese with sliced apple	1 Banana Cinnamon Muffin (page 227) with 1 tablespoon nut butter	Leftover Black Bean & Quinoa Veggie Burger with ½ avocado	Grilled white fish, ½ sweet potato with coconut oil, broccoli
DAY 4 Whey or vegan-based protein shake (see Recommendations, page 284)	1 cup berries with ½ cup plain low-fat yogurt	Spinach salad with any vegetables, salmon, vinegar and oil	Chickpea & Tomato Salad (page 236) with grilled chicken breast
DAY 5 1 Double Chocolate Protein Muffin (page 230)	2 cups air-popped popcorn with coconut oil (no salt)	Homemade egg salad made with mustard, side of raw veggies, almonds	Sautéed Lemon and Garlic Kale (page 270) with leftover grilled chicken breast

INVERTED PYRAMID TYPE MEAL PLAN: WEEK 2			
Breakfast	**Snack**	**Lunch**	**Dinner**
DAY 1 1 cup cottage cheese with tomatoes over a bed of spinach	Apple with 1 table-spoon nut butter	Turkey burger (no bun), raw veggies, salsa with ½ avocado	Curried Meatballs (page 259) over lentils served with a mixed greens salad
DAY 2 1 Double Chocolate Protein Muffin (page 230) and sliced apple	Fresh vegetables with Basic Hummus (page 214)	Leftover Curried Meatballs with mixed greens salad	Kale, mushroom and onion omelet with a side of quinoa
DAY 3 ½ cup plain low-fat yogurt with cinnamon, berries and 2 table-spoons walnuts	1 hard-boiled egg and fresh veggies	Orange & Green Quinoa (page 274) with diced chicken	Savory Sautéed Spinach (page 271) with salmon
DAY 4 Green Goddess Smoothie (page 220)	2 cups air-popped popcorn with coconut oil (no salt)	Spinach salad with any vegetables, chicken breast, vinegar and oil	Grilled chicken breast, ½ sweet potato, broccoli
DAY 5 2 scrambled eggs with spinach & tomato, cooked in coconut oil	Berries plus handful of almonds (no salt)	Leaf lettuce wrap made with leftover grilled chicken breast with veggies	Grilled white fish with ½ cup brown rice with 1 teaspoon coconut oil and 1 cup steamed spinach

INVERTED PYRAMID TYPE MEAL PLAN: WEEK 3			
Breakfast	Snack	Lunch	Dinner
DAY 1 ½ cup oatmeal with 2 tablespoons nut butter and cinnamon (option to add stevia or 1 tablespoon honey)	Green apple with 1 tablespoon nut butter	Black Bean & Tomato Salad (page 234) and guacamole with veggies	Shredded BBQ Chicken (page 254) and Clean Cole Slaw (page 276)
DAY 2 1 Lemon Chia Seed Muffin (page 229) and 1 hard-boiled egg	Basic Hummus (page 214) with fresh vegetables	Leftover Shredded BBQ Chicken and Clean Cole Slaw	Grilled chicken salad with vegetable plus vinegar and olive oil dressing
DAY 3 2 eggs with kale or spinach cooked in coconut oil	2 cups air-popped popcorn with coconut oil (no salt)	1 ½ cups plain low-fat yogurt, 1 cup berries, 2 tablespoons walnuts and cinnamon	Lentil Burger (page 250, no bun), sliced avocado, fresh veggies
DAY 4 Omega Berry Smoothie (page 221)	1 Lemon Chia Seed Muffin (page 229)	Leftover Lentil Burger (no bun) with sliced tomato and avocado	Sweet Potato Turkey Burger (page 262, no bun), mixed greens salad
DAY 5 ½ cup plain low-fat yogurt, berries, cinnamon, 2 tablespoons walnuts	½ cup pumpkin seeds (no salt added) and a green apple	Leftover Sweet Potato Turkey Burger (no bun), fresh vegetables	Grilled white fish, steamed spinach with olive oil, salt, broccoli

INVERTED PYRAMID TYPE MEAL PLAN: WEEK 4

	Breakfast	Snack	Lunch	Dinner
DAY 1	1 Strawberry Muffin (page 233), 1 hard-boiled egg	Blueberry Spinach Smoothie (page 217)	Quinoa Tabouli (page 239) with avocado	Pot Pie Crumble (page 252) and a mixed greens salad
DAY 2	Overnight Chia Seed Oatmeal (page 226) *note:* prepare the night before	Fresh vegetables with Spicy Black Bean Dip (page 278)	Leftover Pot Pie Crumble	One-Pot Turkey Vegetable Chili (page 266)
DAY 3	2 egg spinach & mushroom omelet with diced tomatoes	2 cups air-popped popcorn with coconut oil (no salt)	Leftover One-Pot Turkey Vegetable Chili	Turkey-Stuffed Peppers (page 265)
DAY 4	1 Double Chocolate Protein Muffin (page 230), 1 hard-boiled egg	Apple with 2 tablespoons nut butter	Turkey burger (no cheese) with side salad drizzled with olive oil and vinegar	Grilled chicken salad with vegetable plus vinegar and olive oil dressing
DAY 5	Cinnamon Berry Smoothie (page 212)	1 Double Chocolate Protein Muffin (page 230)	Chopped salad with avocado, egg, tomato, onion, olive oil, vinegar	Grilled salmon and sautéed spinach with brown rice

INVERTED PYRAMID TYPE MEAL PLAN: WEEK 5			
Breakfast	**Snack**	**Lunch**	**Dinner**
DAY 1 2 scrambled eggs and fresh berries	¼ cup unsalted mixed nuts and fresh veggies	Citrus Mint Quinoa Salad (page 237) with diced chicken and avocado	Grilled chicken with steamed vegetables tossed in coconut oil
DAY 2 ½ cup oatmeal and 2 tablespoons walnuts, coconut milk and cinnamon	Avocado Berry Smoothie (page 223)	Leftover Citrus Mint Quinoa Salad with diced chicken and avocado	Southwest Fajita Salad (page 242)
DAY 3 1 cup plain low-fat yogurt with 1 tablespoon chia seeds, berries and cinnamon	Green apple with 2 tablespoons nut butter	Leftover Southwest Fajita Salad	Taco Style Turkey Sloppy Joes (page 264) with ½ sweet potato
DAY 4 Cinnamon Berry Smoothie (page 212)	2 hard-boiled eggs, carrots	Leftover Taco Style Turkey Sloppy Joes with ½ sweet potato	White fish with coconut oil, lemon, sea salt, broccoli
DAY 5 2 hard-boiled eggs, bacon and sliced tomatoes	Spicy Black Bean Dip (page 278) with fresh veggies	Grilled chicken salad with vegetable plus vinegar and olive oil dressing	Black Bean, Corn & Red Pepper Lettuce Wraps (page 246) with ½ avocado

INVERTED PYRAMID TYPE MEAL PLAN: WEEK 6			
Breakfast	**Snack**	**Lunch**	**Dinner**
DAY 1 2 poached eggs over sautéed spinach	Apple with ¼ cup plain low-fat yogurt and cinnamon dip	Simple Butternut Squash Soup (page 272), fresh vegetables, Basic Hummus (page 214)	Cauliflower Crust Pizza (page 248) with mixed greens salad
DAY 2 Creamy Green Dream Smoothie (page 219)	1 Chocolate Chunk Avocado Cookie (page 282)	Napa & Red Cabbage Salad (page 238)	Chicken Vegetable Curry (page 256) with brown rice or quinoa
DAY 3 ½ cup old-fashioned oats with 2 tablespoons walnuts, cinnamon	½ cup berries and 2 tablespoons nut butter	Leftover Chicken Vegetable Curry	Leftover Napa & Red Cabbage Salad with grilled chicken
DAY 4 2 hard-boiled eggs, 1 cup fresh berries	2 No Bake Chocolate Energy Balls (page 281)	Rainbow Kale Salad (page 240) with grilled chicken	Split Pea & Turkey Soup (page 273)
DAY 5 1 Oat & Almond Breakfast Bar (page 225) with 1 tablespoon honey	½ cup low-fat yogurt with berries and cinnamon	Leftover Split Pea & Turkey Soup	Roasted Parsnips & Carrots (page 275) with salmon

Eat Right for Your Hourglass Type

Control your health and your weight with this simple plan. You'll have to steer clear of dairy, coffee and heavy meats, but you'll be able to indulge in a healthy amount of complex carbohydrates; clean, lean meats and warm spices stoke the furnace that is your metabolism.

HOURGLASS TYPE EATING PLAN CHEAT SHEET	
Eat This	**Cut Back or Eliminate This**
Raw Vegetables, Fruits & Salads, Juices: Mixed greens salads, low-glycemic fruits	*Dairy:* Creams, cheeses, ice cream, yogurt, etc. (eliminate entirely)
Complex Carbohydrates: Old-fashioned oats, quinoa, brown rice	*Heavy Meats:* High-fat red meats, dark meat poultry
Warm Spices: Cinnamon, cumin, turmeric, curry, red pepper	*Caffeine:* Coffee, black tea, cola/diet cola (eliminate entirely)
Lean Meats: Eggs, turkey and chicken breast, lean cuts of pork, white fish	*Refined Carbohydrates:* White bread, pastries, cookies, pasta

Hourglass Type Eating Plan Basics Shopping List

Here is a basic Hourglass Type shopping list with just the staples. Add on as you see fit based on the meals or snacks you plan on making throughout the week.

- Apples
- Avocados
- Berries (fresh and frozen)
- Broccoli
- Brown rice
- Brussels sprouts
- Cauliflower
- Chia seeds
- Coconut oil
- Garlic
- Leafy greens (spinach, romaine, kale)
- Lean ground turkey (organic preferred)
- Nut butter
- Nuts (almonds, walnuts, etc.)
- Old-fashioned oatmeal
- Olive oil
- Omega-3 fatty acids (see Recommendations, page 284)
- Onions
- Organic chicken breasts
- Organic eggs
- Probiotics (see Recommendations, page 284)
- Protein powder (see Recommendations, page 284)
- Prunes
- Quinoa
- Salmon*
- Tomatoes
- White fish, such as cod, tilapia and halibut

Even though salmon is a higher-fat fish, it's full of heart-healthy omega-3 fatty acids. Omega-3 fatty acids are something we all need more of.

HOURGLASS TYPE MEAL PLAN: WEEK 1

	Breakfast	Snack	Lunch	Dinner
DAY 1	2 eggs over black beans with tomatoes and onions	Generous handful of almonds or walnuts	Grilled salmon salad with fresh or grilled vegetables	Spaghetti Squash with Turkey Bolognese (page 260) with small side salad
DAY 2	½ cup oatmeal with coconut milk, cinnamon and 2 tablespoons walnuts	Fresh vegetables with 2 tablespoons guacamole and salsa	Leftover Spaghetti Squash with Turkey Bolognese with small side salad	Black Bean & Quinoa Veggie Burgers (page 247) with broccoli
DAY 3	2 eggs over black beans with tomatoes and onions	Apple with 1 tablespoon nut butter	Leftover Black Bean & Quinoa Veggie Burgers with carrots	Grilled white fish, ½ sweet potato with coconut oil, broccoli
DAY 4	Whey or vegan-based protein shake (see Recommendations, page 284)	2 tablespoons Spicy Black Bean Dip (page 278) with fresh vegetables	Spinach salad with any vegetables, chicken breast, vinegar and oil	Black Bean, Corn & Red Pepper Lettuce Wraps (page 246) with salsa
DAY 5	Cinnamon Berry Smoothie (page 212)	2 cups air-popped popcorn with coconut oil (no salt)	Homemade egg salad made with mustard, side of raw veggies, almonds	Sautéed Lemon and Garlic Kale (page 270) with grilled chicken breast

HOURGLASS TYPE MEAL PLAN: WEEK 2			
Breakfast	**Snack**	**Lunch**	**Dinner**
DAY 1 Chia Berry Smoothie (page 218)	Hard-boiled egg with vegetables	Turkey burger (no bun), raw veggies, salsa and ½ avocado	Curried Meatballs (page 259) over lentils served with a mixed greens salad
DAY 2 1 Quinoa Protein Power Muffin (page 232) and 1 hard-boiled egg	Fresh vegetables with Basic Hummus (page 214)	Leftover Curried Meatballs with mixed greens salad	Kale, mushroom and onion omelet with a side of quinoa
DAY 3 ½ cup old-fashioned oats with cinnamon, berries and 2 table-spoons chia seeds	1 Chocolate Coconut Energy Muffin (page 228)	Orange and Green Quinoa (page 274) with diced chicken	Savory Sautéed Spinach (page 271) with salmon
DAY 4 Avocado Berry Smoothie (page 223)	2 cups air-popped popcorn with coconut oil (no salt)	Spinach salad with any vegetables, chicken breast, vinegar and oil	Grilled chicken breast, ½ sweet potato, broccoli
DAY 5 2 hard-boiled eggs with sliced apple	5 prunes plus handful of raw nuts	Leaf lettuce wrap made with leftover grilled chicken breast with veggies and salsa	Orange & Green Quinoa (page 274) with grilled white fish

HOURGLASS TYPE MEAL PLAN: WEEK 3

	Breakfast	Snack	Lunch	Dinner
DAY 1	½ cup old-fashioned oatmeal with 2 tablespoons chia seeds and cinnamon	Green apple with 1 tablespoon nut butter	Black Bean & Tomato Salad (page 234) and fresh veggies	Shredded BBQ Chicken (page 254) and Clean Cole Slaw (page 276)
DAY 2	1 Lemon Chia Seed Muffin (page 229) and 1 hard-boiled egg	Basic Hummus (page 214) with fresh vegetables	Leftover Shredded BBQ Chicken and Clean Cole Slaw	Grilled chicken salad with vegetable plus vinegar and olive oil dressing
DAY 3	½ cup old-fashioned oatmeal with 1 tablespoon unsweetened nut butter and cinnamon	2 cups air-popped popcorn with coconut oil (no salt)	Turkey burger (no cheese or bun) with steamed vegetables	Lentil Burger (page 250, no bun), sliced avocado, fresh veggies
DAY 4	Cinnamon Berry Smoothie (page 212)	1 Lemon Chia Seed Muffin (page 229)	Leftover Lentil Burger (no bun) with sliced tomato and avocado	Sweet Potato Turkey Burger (page 262), mixed greens salad
DAY 5	2 hard-boiled eggs with fresh berries	Fresh veggies and Spicy Black Bean Dip (page 278)	Leftover Sweet Potato Turkey Burger (no bun), fresh vegetables	Grilled white fish, steamed spinach with olive oil, salt, broccoli

HOURGLASS TYPE MEAL PLAN: WEEK 4

	Breakfast	Snack	Lunch	Dinner
DAY 1	1 Strawberry Muffin (page 233), 1 hard-boiled egg	Blueberry Spinach Smoothie (page 217)	Quinoa Tabouli (page 239) with avocado	Pot Pie Crumble (page 252) and a mixed greens salad
DAY 2	Overnight Chia Seed Oatmeal (page 226) *note:* prepare the night before	1 Strawberry Muffin (page 233)	Leftover Pot Pie Crumble	One-Pot Turkey Vegetable Chili (page 266)
DAY 3	2 egg spinach & mushroom omelet with diced tomatoes	Fresh vegetables with Spicy Black Bean Dip (page 278)	Leftover One-Pot Turkey Vegetable Chili	Turkey-Stuffed Peppers (page 265)
DAY 4	1 Double Chocolate Protein Muffin (page 230) and fresh berries	5 prunes plus small handful of almonds	Leftover Turkey-Stuffed Peppers	Grilled chicken salad with vegetable plus vinegar and olive oil dressing
DAY 5	Avocado Berry Smoothie (page 223)	1 Double Chocolate Protein Muffin (page 230)	Chopped salad with avocado, egg, tomato, onion, olive oil, vinegar and sea salt	Grilled salmon and sautéed spinach with brown rice

HOURGLASS TYPE MEAL PLAN: WEEK 5

	Breakfast	Snack	Lunch	Dinner
DAY 1	2 scrambled eggs and fresh berries	Unsalted mixed nuts and fresh veggies	Citrus Mint Quinoa Salad (page 237) with diced chicken and avocado	Grilled chicken with steamed vegetables tossed in coconut oil
DAY 2	Oatmeal plus 2 tablespoons walnuts, fresh berries and cinnamon	1 hard-boiled egg and sliced apple	Leftover Citrus Mint Quinoa Salad with fresh veggies and Spicy Black Bean Dip (page 278)	Southwest Fajita Salad (page 242)
DAY 3	1 Banana Cinnamon Muffin (page 227) with berries	Avocado Berry Smoothie (page 223)	Leftover Southwest Fajita Salad	Taco Style Turkey Sloppy Joes (page 264) with ½ sweet potato
DAY 4	Avocado Berry Smoothie (page 223)	5 prunes plus small handful of almonds	Black Bean, Corn & Red Pepper Lettuce Wraps (page 246) with ½ avocado	2 egg omelet with ½ cup quinoa and steamed vegetables
DAY 5	2 hard-boiled eggs and fresh berries	Spicy Black Bean Dip (page 278) with fresh veggies	Grilled chicken salad with vegetable plus vinegar and olive oil dressing	White fish with coconut oil, lemon, sea salt, broccoli

HOURGLASS TYPE MEAL PLAN: WEEK 6			
Breakfast	**Snack**	**Lunch**	**Dinner**
DAY 1 ¼ cup old-fashioned oats and 2 tablespoons chia seeds with cinnamon and berries	2 cups air-popped popcorn with coconut oil (no salt)	Simple Butternut Squash Soup (page 272) with side salad with vinegar and olive oil	Grilled white fish with steamed broccoli with coconut oil
DAY 2 Cinnamon Berry Smoothie (page 212)	1 Chocolate Chunk Avocado Cookie (page 282)	Napa & Red Cabbage Salad (page 238)	Chicken Vegetable Curry (page 256) with brown rice or quinoa
DAY 3 ½ cup old-fashioned oats with cinnamon and 1 tablespoon unsweetened nut butter	5 prunes plus hard-boiled egg	Leftover Chicken Vegetable Curry	Leftover Napa & Red Cabbage Salad with grilled chicken
DAY 4 2 hard-boiled eggs, fresh berry salad	2 No Bake Chocolate Energy Balls (page 281)	Rainbow Kale Salad (page 240) with grilled chicken	Split Pea & Turkey Soup (page 273)
DAY 5 1 Oat & Almond Breakfast Bar (page 225) with sliced apple	1 hard-boiled egg plus carrots	Leftover Split Pea & Turkey Soup	Roasted Parsnips & Carrots (page 275) with salmon

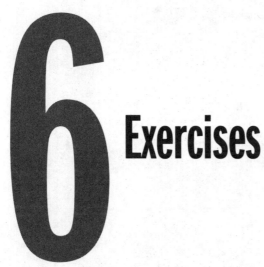

6 Exercises

"*The Belly Burn Plan* helped me transform my body. My middle has always been a problem area for me, and *The Belly Burn Plan* was just what I needed. The exercise plan doesn't take a lot of time or equipment, and the workouts are fantastic."

—CINDY B., AGE 52

All of the workouts in this book include exercises appropriate for your fitness level, some of which you may not be familiar with. In this chapter, you'll find easy-to-follow definitions of the exercises, many of which include photo demonstrations. Not only will you be in great shape by the end of the program, you'll be fitness savvy, too.

Equipment

You'll be amazed by the number of exercises you'll do in *The Belly Burn Plan* that require absolutely no additional equipment at all. The most frequently used piece of equipment you'll use is your own body. Beyond that, the most you'll need is a set of hand-held weights, like dumbbells. If you don't have access to dumbbells, get creative. Lots of household items can be substituted for dumbbells, including:

- Books
- Gallons of Water
- Pans/Pots (with handles)
- Soup/Vegetable Cans

The weight of the dumbbells or hand-held weights you choose to use depends on the strength of different muscles. Generally speaking, if you can perform twelve to fifteen repetitions of any exercise with ease using one particular weight, it's time to bump it up. On the other hand, if you're having a problem making it to twelve repetitions because the weight feels too heavy, it's best to drop down a pound or two.

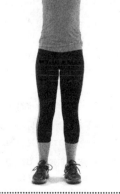

Arm Circles:

1. Usually done with no weight at all, extend your arms straight out from your sides.
2. Without bending your elbows, make small, tight circles with your arms. Don't let your arms drop.
3. Continue making circles until your set is complete.

Arm Circles

Back Extension:

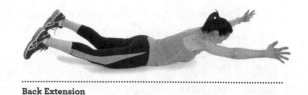

Back Extension

1. Start by lying face down on the ground with your arms and legs extended out in a V, nose pointed down.
2. Pull your arms and legs off the ground. Concentrate on pulling your shoulder blades back while squeezing your bottom to help maintain the position.

Tip: To maintain the proper form, keep your nose pointed down to the ground. Squeeze your bottom as you bring your arms and legs off the ground.

Bicep Curls:

1. Holding a handheld weight in each hand, bring your arms to a 90 degree angle with your palms facing up.
2. Keeping your elbows in at your sides, slowly raise the weights bringing your palms toward your shoulders.
3. After your palms are up toward your shoulders, release them slowly back down to the starting position without moving your elbows from your sides.

Body Weight Squats:

1. Stand with your legs shoulder-width apart.
2. Drop down by bending your knees, as if you're going to sit into a chair.
3. Return to a standing position.

Tip: Try to get your thighs as parallel to the floor as possible. Focus on keeping your shoulders pointed up toward the ceiling, getting your bottom back as far as possible and keeping your knees over your toes. Draw your abs in through the entire exercise and squeeze your bottom on the way up.

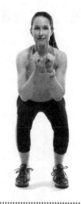

Body Weight Squats

Bridge:

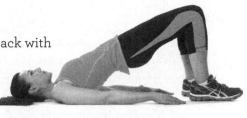

1. Start by lying flat on your back with your knees bent and hands resting at your sides.
2. Push your hips up toward the ceiling, keeping your feet firmly planted.

Bridge

Tip: Squeeze your glutes (bottom) and try to prevent your hips from dropping. If you look down at your body toward your knees, you should be able to clearly see your hips and thighs. Hold this position for the designated period of time.

Broad Jumps:

1. Standing with your feet shoulder-width apart, drop down into a squat position.
2. Spring *forward*, jumping as far as possible. Land softly by bending your knees and absorbing the jump. Turn around and repeat.

Tip: Never lock your knees. To get as much distance out of your jump, look well beyond the point where you think you might land. Visually "overshoot" your goal.

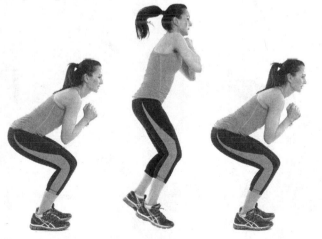

Broad Jumps

Burpees:

1. Start by standing with your feet shoulder-width apart.
2. In one motion, drop down into a squat, reach forward and plant your hands on the ground in front of your feet.
3. Without moving your hands, kick your feet back so you're in a straight-arm plank position.
4. As soon as your body is planked out, return to position 2.
5. Jump straight up, allowing your feet to leave the ground.

To do half burpees:

1. Start in a straight-arm plank position (Burpee step 3).
2. Jump your legs in, tucking your knees under your chest, finishing in a squat position (Burpee step 4).
3. Jump back into a straight-arm plank position and repeat.

Tip: This exercise is tough but well worth it! You'll work all the muscles in your body and your lungs, too.

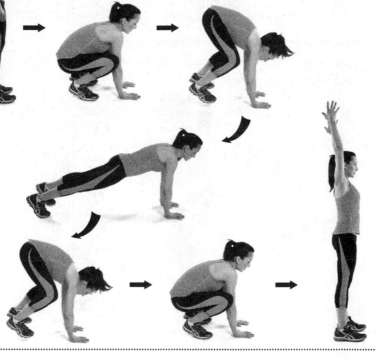

Burpees

Calf Raises:

1. Start by standing with your feet flat, spaced just a few inches apart. Lift your heels off the ground, coming up to the balls of your feet.
2. Bring heels back down to the ground, repeating this up/down motion continuously.

Tip: The muscles in your calves are important, but smaller than some of the other muscles through your thighs and bottom. Expect your calves to feel as if they're on fire as you reach the end of each set.

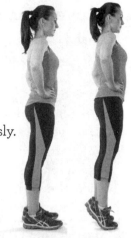

Calf Raises

Clock Lunges:

These lunges bring your legs to the twelve o'clock, three o'clock and six o'clock position in five easy steps.

1. Step forward into a traditional lunge position, moving your forward leg to twelve o'clock.
2. Return to standing.
3. Step out to a side lunge at three o'clock.
4. Return to standing.
5. Take a big step back doing a reverse lunge to six o'clock.

Tip: Each set is one clock lunge. The opposite foot of the leg that's doing the lunging stays in the same spot with the exception of a slight pivot.

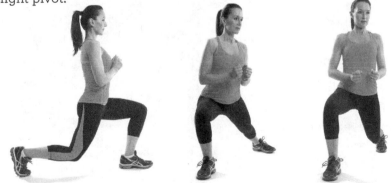

Foward Lunge   **Side Lunge**   **Reverse Lunge**

Crossover Punches:

1. Stand with your feet shoulder-width apart and arms bent holding two hand-held weights.
2. Punch across your body to the opposite side, holding your abs in as tight as possible. Your arm should finish straight with your palm facing down toward the ground.
3. Draw your arm back into the starting position and repeat on the opposite side, alternating continuously.

Tip: Keep a slight bend in your knees and don't forget to use your abs. Think of driving your fist into a punching bag before bringing it back to repeat on the opposite side.

Crossover Punches

Curtsy Squats:

1. Start with your feet shoulder-width apart.
2. Step one leg back and across the opposite leg, like a curtsy, then squat down.
3. Come back to a standing position and repeat on the opposite side.

Tip: This exercise works the sides of the hips, helping to shape and tone your bottom. Your backside will thank you later!

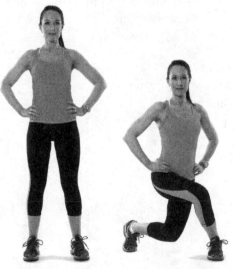

Curtsy Squats

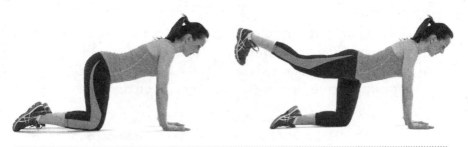

Donkey Kicks

Donkey Kicks:

1. Start by resting on your hands and knees in a tabletop position. Keep your neck relaxed with your nose pointed down at the ground.
2. Take one leg, and kick it straight behind you, pushing through your heel.
3. Bring the leg back toward your belly and repeat on the opposite side.

Tip: Your hands don't move and your hips should stay square. Remember to draw your abs in toward your spine.

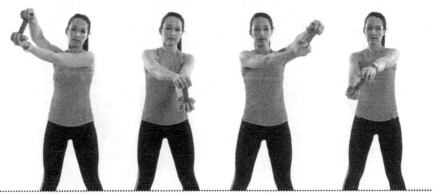

Figure-8 Shoulder Sizzler

Figure-8 Shoulder Sizzler:

Use a hand-held weight (ideally between 5 and 10 pounds) for this exercise.

1. Stand with your feet hip-width apart, toes pointed forward and a slight bend in your knees.

2. Hold the weight with both hands and raise your arms so they're at shoulder height and directly in front of you.
3. Draw your abs in and start moving the weight into a large, horizontal figure eight (or infinity sign, if you prefer).

Tip: This exercise works your shoulders and your abs. Keep your elbows locked and belly button drawn in and be sure not to move your hips or feet. You don't need a lot of weight for this exercise, but don't be afraid to upgrade a pound or two if you're not feeling it after the first set.

Heel Taps:

1. Lie flat on the ground with your knees bent.
2. Extend your arms down toward your feet and raise your head and shoulders off the ground.
3. Tap your right hand against your right heel, then your left hand against your left heel.
4. Keep your head and shoulders off the ground until all repetitions are complete.

Tip: Pull your belly button toward your spine and lower back toward the ground.

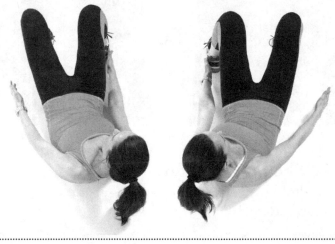

Heel Taps

Hip Dips:

1. Start this exercise by turning on your side, resting on your forearm with your elbow bent.
2. Stack your feet on top of one another.
3. Push your hips up, then drop them back down to the ground.

Tip: To avoid rolling forward, keep your free hand off the ground and resting on your hip or along the side of your leg.

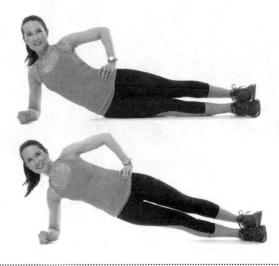

Hip Dips

High Knee Running:
Think marching-band knees, just a little higher and faster!

1. Simply jog or march in place, pulling your knees as high as possible.

Tip: Keep your body straight, abs tight and pull your knees as close to your chest as possible.

Note: Beginner workouts perform a variation of High Knee Running called High Knee Marching. Your heart rate will still get a boost without all the impact. To perform the exercise, simply pull your knees up to your chest at a walking pace.

Inchworms:

1. Start by standing straight, then bend over and touch the ground. Bend your knees, only if necessary.
2. Slowly walk your hands forward until your body is completely planked out.
3. Without moving your hands, slowly walk your feet forward until they meet your hands.
4. After completing one inchworm, keep moving, walking your hands out, followed by your feet.

   Tip: Be sure to keep your belly button pulled into your spine to support your lower back.

Inchworms

Lateral Arm Raises:

1. Start by holding a light weight in each hand at your sides.
2. With a slight bend in your elbows, raise your arms out from your sides up to shoulder height.
3. Slowly return back to the starting position.

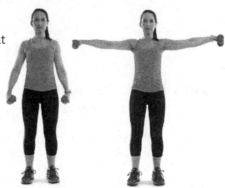

Lateral Arm Raises

Tip: If you extend beyond your shoulders, much of the effort is lost. Do each repetition slowly, with extra attention paid to how high you lift your arms. This is a great exercise for the small muscles of the shoulders that helps to give a lot of definition.

Lunge & Twists:

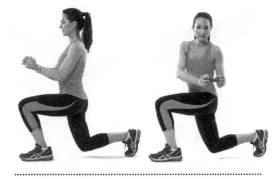

1. Start by stepping into a traditional lunge position.
2. When your body has reached a comfortable forward position, extend your arms forward holding one weight with both hands, then twist your body in the direction of your *lead* leg.

Lunge & Twists

3. Return to a standing position and repeat, alternating sides.

Tip: When you step out and lunge on your left leg, use the weight and twist to your left side. Do the same, but twisting to your right, when you're leading with your right leg.

Lunges:

1. Start by standing with your feet about hip-width apart.
2. Step one foot out about two to three feet in front of you.
3. Bending your front knee, and dropping your back knee closer to the ground, enter a lunge position.
4. Keep your back straight and don't let your front knee extend beyond your toes.
5. Return to a standing position. Alternate legs, or repeat continuously on the same leg.

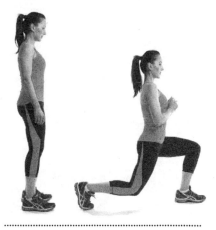

Tip: Avoid the mistake of leaning forward over your knees. Protect your knees and keep your shoulders in line with your hips.

Lunges

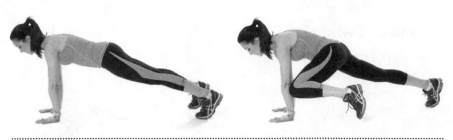

Mountain Climbers

Mountain Climbers:

1. Start down on the ground in a straight-arm plank position, resting on your hands and toes with your back straight.
2. Bring your right knee up and in toward your right elbow.
3. Return your right foot back to the starting position.
4. Repeat on the opposite side by bringing your left knee to your left elbow.

Tip: Concentrate on keeping your abs drawn in and pulling your knee as close as possible to your elbow. This is a great full-body exercise that gives extra attention to your abs, back and shoulders.

Oblique Twists:

This exercise can be done with any weighted object (ideally between 5 and 10 pounds) that you can hold firmly with both hands, such as a dumbbell, medicine ball or even a gallon of water.

1. Start by sitting with your knees bent and heels planted on the ground.
2. Slowly lean back until you feel your abs engage.

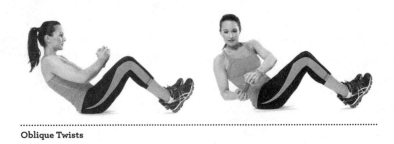

Oblique Twists

3. Move the weight in a twisting motion from the right hip to the left hip, getting as high of an arch as possible.

Tip: If your core is strong enough, lift your heels off the ground to perform this exercise. Twist your body from your shoulders to your waist while keeping your belly button pulled to your spine.

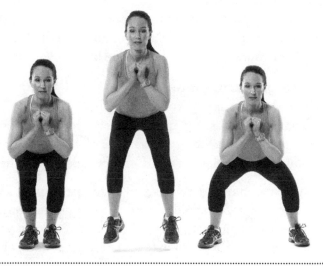

Out & Ins

Out & Ins:

1. To begin, stand in a squat-like position, feet about six inches apart.
2. Jump both feet out, finishing in a wide-leg squat position (this is your "out").
3. Hop both feet back in to your starting position (this is your "in").

Tip: Always stay in your squat. Don't stand up! Your legs deserve the workout.

Plank:

This exercise can be done one of two ways, either as a traditional forearm plank or as a straight-arm plank.

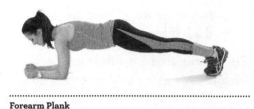

Forearm Plank

To do a forearm plank:

1. Start by lying face down on the ground.
2. Resting on your forearms, push your body off the ground with the rest of your core supported by the balls of your feet or toes.

To do a straight-arm plank:

1. Start on your hands and knees.
2. Keep your hands resting under your shoulders and extend your legs straight back, resting on the balls of your feet or toes.
3. Maintain this position for the duration called for in the workout.

Tip: If you're just beginning, you may need to rest on your knees. As you get stronger, try to avoid resting on your knees altogether. Regardless of the position you're in, it's important to keep your back straight, neck in a neutral position (avoid drooping) and pelvis tucked under to protect your back.

Plank & Row:

1. Start in a straight-arm plank position.
2. With your right arm, row a dumbbell (between 8 to 15 pounds) up, pulling your elbow toward the ceiling.
3. Return weight to the ground and repeat with your left arm, alternating sides continuously.

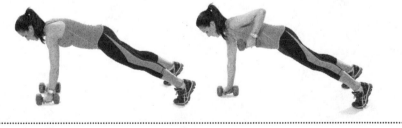

Plank & Row

Tip: Try to keep your abs as tight as possible and use the heaviest weight you can manage. Keep your hips level to the ground, and make sure all the motion comes from your arm.

Plank Jacks:

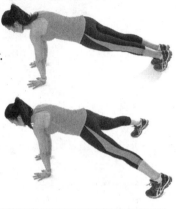

1. Start in a straight-arm plank position with your feet close together.
2. Like a horizontal jumping jack, jump your feet out into a wide V position without moving your upper body.
3. Quickly jump your feet back together to the starting position.

Tip: Don't forget, this is still an abs exercise, so keep your tummy tight the entire time.

Plank Jacks

Plank to Push-Ups:

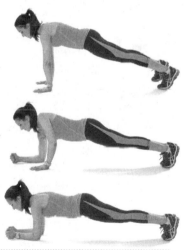

1. Start this exercise in a straight-arm plank position.
2. Drop down to your right forearm (left hand stays in place).
3. Drop down to your left forearm (ending in a forearm plank position).
4. Push up onto your right hand (left arm stays in place).
5. Push up onto your left hand (ending in a straight arm plank position).

Plank to Push-Ups

This is *one* repetition. Continue the exercises by dropping down one arm at a time, then pushing up one arm at a time. Be sure to alternate sides.

Tip: Keep your abs tight and try to stay off your knees as much as possible. This is a great exercise for the shoulders, chest, back and abs.

Plié Squats:

1. Begin by standing in a modified plié position (with your heels about hip-width apart and toes pointed out at a 45-degree angle).
2. Drop your hips down as deep as possible while pushing your knees out to the sides. Hold for one second.
3. Return to the standing position, squeezing your bottom, and pull up on your toes to keep the weight over your heels.

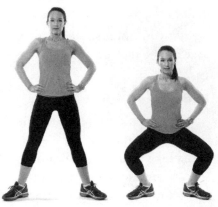

Plié Squats

Tip: This exercise not only works the quadriceps of the top of the thighs, but also the abductor and adductor muscles of the outer and inner thighs.

Plyo Jumps:

1. Start with your feet hip-width apart.
2. Squat deeply.
3. Come out of the squat by jumping as high as you can, leading with your arms.
4. As you come down, land as softly as possible, bending your knees to absorb the jump.

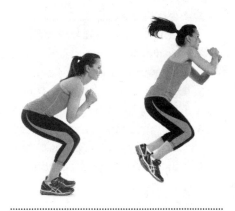

Plyo Jumps

Tip: This exercise works the big muscles of your thighs and bottom. Because Plyo Jumps push your heart rate up high and fast, the number of repetitions is fairly low. Do every Plyo Jump slowly and controlled, focusing on the quality of the jump, rather than how fast you can get through it.

Reverse Fly:

1. Start by standing with your back straight, holding a light set of dumbbells, one in each hand.
2. Bend over to a 45-degree angle and allow your arms to drop softly in front of you.
3. With your belly button pulled back toward your spine, open your arms out wide, like the wings of a bird.
4. Slowly drop your arms and bring them back in toward the center of your body.

Tip: You should be able to see the weights in your peripheral vision. If you can't, your arms are too far back. This is an excellent exercise for the shoulders and back.

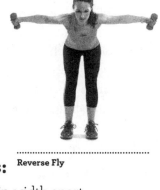

Reverse Fly

Reverse Lunge to Forward Kicks:

1. Start by standing with your feet about hip-width apart.
2. Take a big step *back* with one leg and drop down into a reverse lunge.
3. From the reverse lunge position, kick the back leg forward, straight out in front of you, driving with your heel, pulling your toes to your face.
4. Go immediately into the next reverse lunge alternating legs continuously.

Tip: Lunges are great for working all the muscles through the thighs, hips and bottom. You'll also improve your balance and push your heart rate up by driving your leg forward into a powerful kick.

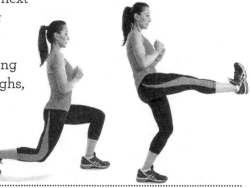

Reverse Lunge to Forward Kicks

Scissor Kicks:

1. Start by lying on your back with your hands tucked under your back at your tailbone, palms down.
2. Firmly press your lower back down into the ground.
3. Without bending your knees, slowly lift your legs between 30 and 45 degrees off the ground in a V position.
4. Crisscross your legs over one another, pointing your toes away from you the entire time.

Tip: This is an incredible exercise for your abs. For more of a challenge, hover your feet as close as possible to the ground without making contact.

Scissor Kicks

Shoulder Press:

1. Holding a set of dumbbells that are a heavy weight, but something you can manage, stand with your feet shoulder-width apart and your knees slightly bent.
2. Bend your elbows and raise your arms, starting with the weights just above ear level.
3. Push the weights up toward the ceiling until your arms straighten out.
4. Slowly return the weights to the starting bent position and repeat.

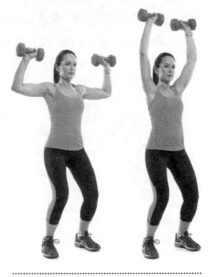

Shoulder Press

Tip: This exercise primarily works the big muscles of the shoulders, but is supported by the biceps (top of the upper arm) and triceps (the back of the upper arm) as well.

Shoulder Press Squats:

1. Using a set of dumbbells that are a challenging weight, but something you can manage, begin this exercise like a traditional shoulder press.
2. As your arms come down from the top position of the shoulder press, drop down into as deep of a squat as possible.
3. As you come out of the squat, drive your arms back up overhead into a shoulder press.

Tip: This is an efficient combination exercise that works the big muscles of the shoulders while getting into the hips, thighs and bottom, too. Always remember to squeeze your bottom and draw in your abs throughout the entire exercise.

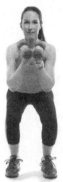

Shoulder Press Squats

Side Plank:

1. Start by sitting with your legs extended over to one side.
2. Place your hand on the ground, just under your shoulder. Keep the weight on your hand equally distributed from fingertips to palm.
3. With your legs extended, stack your feet on top of each other, push your hips up and raise the opposite arm up into the air—reaching for the sky. Now hold.

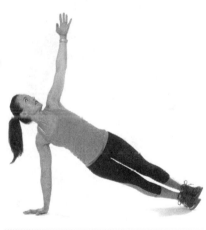

Side Plank

Tip: You have the option to stagger your feet if you can't quite manage to stack them on top of each other. This is a great exercise for working the oblique muscles of the abs as well as the stabilizing muscles of the shoulders.

Split Leg Squats:

1. Start by facing forward and placing one foot up on a bench or a chair behind you, resting on your toes. Your legs should be split, similar to a lunge position.
2. Without changing the position of the leg behind you, bend your front knee into a single leg squat position, keeping your back straight and abs tight.

Tip: Make sure your knee does not extend over your toes when dropping into the single leg squat position. If it does, slowly hop the leg forward a couple of inches.

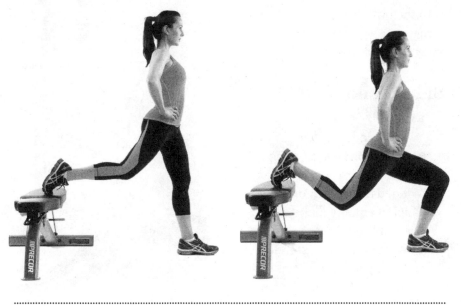

Split Leg Squats

Squat Jumps:

1. Stand with your feet hip-width apart.
2. Bend your knees and drop into a squat position with your thighs as close to parallel with the ground as possible. Think of sitting into a chair as you come down.
3. As soon as you drop down into this position, spring back up, jumping off the ground a few inches. Land by bending your knees and dropping back into the next Squat Jump.

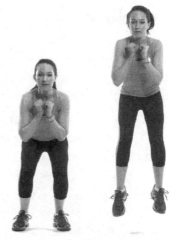

Squat Jumps

Tip: Squat Jumps are a faster, less intense version of Plyo Jumps. The goal is to get in a high number of repetitions with less of a lift off the ground.

Squat to Side Kicks:

1. Start with your feet shoulder-width apart.
2. Drop down into a squat position.
3. As you come to a stand, kick one leg out to the side, driving your leg out until it is as close to horizontal as possible.

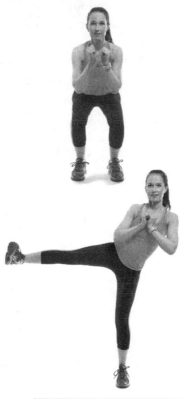

Tip: Pull your toes toward your face, aiming with your heel. Drop down to a squat and repeat on the opposite side.

Squat to Side Kicks

Step-Ups:

This exercise should be done with a sturdy bench, step or riser that is about knee height. Lower is okay, but higher is not. A step that is too high could lead to a knee injury.

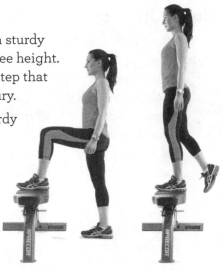

1. Place your right foot on a sturdy bench, step or riser. Step up.
2. Drop back down onto the ground, holding the right foot on the step until the number of repetitions for that leg is complete.
3. Switch to the left leg, placing your left foot on the step.

Step-Ups

Tricep Dips:

1. Sit on the edge of a sturdy bench, step or riser with the palms of your hands grasping the edge of the seat at the outside of your thighs.
2. With your arms as straight as possible, walk your bottom off the seat, suspending your upper body with your hands only.
3. Keep your knees bent and slowly bend your elbows behind you.
4. Return to the straight-arm position before dipping back down to a bent arm position. Repeat continuously until set is complete.

Tip: This exercise works the triceps in the back of the arms. These muscles are small and usually much weaker than the bigger shoulder and bicep muscles. The closer your feet are to the edge of the seat, the easier the exercise is. The farther you walk them out, the more difficult it becomes.

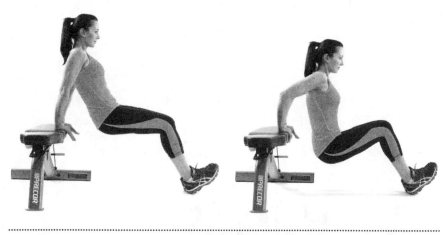

Tricep Dips

Wall Squat:

1. Lean against a wall with your feet hip-width apart and about sixteen inches out from the wall.
2. Drop your hips down to the point that it looks as though you're sitting in a chair.

Tip: Don't let your knees collapse in. Your knees should not be over your toes, so adjust your feet if needed.

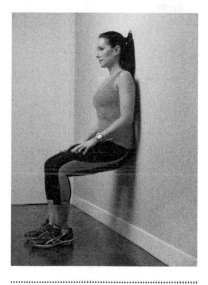

Wall Squat

7 Workouts

"I have to say these workouts are really pushing me and I am doing the beginner level! The most exercise I have done in many years is walking my dogs, which is also a challenge. Thank you!"

—LINDA N., AGE 58

Are you ready to push your heart rate up and get your muscles moving? You're about to start in on twenty-two full-body high-intensity interval workouts that will tone and shape your body from head to toe. Remember, high-intensity workouts are tough, but done at *your* fitness level.

By selecting the workout level most appropriate for your body (Beginner, Intermediate, Advanced), you'll see significant improvements by the end of the program. As you progress through the workout plan, so will your fitness level. The goal of the workouts is to get you in the habit of exercising three to four times a week. Often, all it takes is thirty-five minutes to boost your metabolism, increase energy and burn fat.

All of the workouts are between thirty and sixty minutes. Some are strength-focused, some are cardio-focused and some are a combination of the two. All of the workouts are designed to get your body moving in a way that recruits every major muscle group. No two workouts are the same. *The Belly Burn Plan* is the cure for workout boredom.

Determine Your Workout Level

Not sure which level of workout you should follow? A detailed description is given in Chapter 2 on page 22, but here's a recap:

- **Beginner:** If it's been a few months since you last worked out, you're just getting off the couch, or you're new to structured workouts, this is the level for you. The *Beginner*-level exercises will allow your joints to adjust and muscles to develop in a way that will help you grow stronger each and every day. After you finish the twenty-two workouts at the *Beginner* level, you'll be ready to start the workouts all over again, at the *Intermediate* level.
- **Intermediate:** You're familiar with most of the exercises, but don't get to the gym as often as you like, or perhaps you don't push yourself as hard as you think you could. You're ready to dive in at a pace you can handle, while getting your body in incredible shape. All *Intermediate* workouts are a slightly dialed-down version of the *Advanced* workouts . . . a level you'll be ready to jump into after you finish the twenty-two workouts at this level.

- **Advanced:** You know your fitness and your body is up for the challenge! The *Advanced* workouts will be a physical *and* mental challenge for you, improving the strong base of muscular and cardiovascular fitness you have developed. The beauty of *The Belly Burn Plan* workouts is variety. After you wrap up one cycle of the *Advanced* workouts, do them again. Push your pace, get faster and become stronger. The sky is the limit.

Workout Structure

Every workout begins with a warm-up between five and ten minutes. It's important to take this time to loosen up as the intervals you're about to do will put your muscles and joints to the test. Taking a few minutes to get your blood flowing through your body will help ensure you'll stay free of unwanted injury.

Circuits

All of the workouts vary between two and four circuits. The number of times you repeat a circuit is noted at the top of the circuit you're about to begin. Follow the circuits in the order in which they're designed and give 100 percent effort with every exercise. At the end of the circuit, you'll rest for somewhere between one and two minutes. This is also noted at the top of the circuit.

Reps (Repetitions)

Reps are the number of times you perform one specific exercise. For instance, if the workout calls for fifteen shoulder presses, you're instructed to do fifteen repetitions of a shoulder press.

Sets

A set is the number of times you go through each prescribed exercise. The top of every circuit will give you the number of sets you're supposed to do. Let's say a circuit is repeated a total of three times. That means that you're going to do three sets of each exercise.

Rests

Every workout will have a specific amount of time for resting in between circuits. Even if you don't think you need the rest, take it. The workouts become progressively challenging and you don't want to fatigue before the end.

Easy, Moderate and Intense Cardio Zones

You'll notice most of the workouts have you perform easy, moderate or intense cardio for varying periods of time. Varying the intensity of your workout is crucial to *The Belly Burn Plan*, and to your success, so it's important that you understand what the levels mean. Really, it's quite simple. Here is an explanation:

- **Easy Cardio** is exactly what it sounds like—cardiovascular exercise done at an easy pace, similar to something you'd do at the very beginning of a warm-up. At the end of an easy cardio interval, you should feel comfortable enough that you're ready for more exercise. On a scale of 1 to 10, with 10 being the hardest you could push yourself, your effort level is between 1 and 4.
- **Moderate Cardio** picks up the effort slightly from the easy cardio zone. I like to think of this zone as *comfortably uncomfortable*. You're breathing harder, but not breathless. If you wanted to, you could hold this zone for a long period of time. At the end of a moderate cardio interval, you should feel as if you've done a good amount of work, but still have more fuel in the tank. Your effort level is somewhere between 5 and 7.
- **Intense Cardio** is where the magic happens. As far as cardio intervals go, anytime you see Intense Cardio in a workout, you know you're about to do a high-intensity cardiovascular interval. In this zone, you'll push your heart rate up high and begin feeling breathless. The length of time you can hold this zone is short, but don't forget to push yourself. After the end of an Intense Cardio interval, you should feel as if you've given everything you've got. Your effort level is somewhere between 8 and 10.

I can't emphasize enough how important it is to push yourself, physically *and* mentally out of your comfort zone. After just a few weeks, you will *see* and *feel* a difference in your body.

Alternatives to Running or Jogging

The cardio intervals in *The Belly Burn Plan* were designed so you can do them anywhere. If you can't or don't like to run or jog, don't worry! There are a lot of other options. Here are a few suggestions:

- Climb stairs or use a stair climber
- Jog or run outside or on a treadmill
- Ride a stationary bike
- Use an elliptical
- Swim
- Use a rowing machine

Frequency of Workouts

As mentioned earlier, you'll work out three to four times a week. Workouts are structured every other day, for a total of twenty-two sessions in all. Make the most of them by giving 100 percent. Try your best to do the workouts every other day, avoiding back-to-back days. This will allow your body to recover enough to give all you've got for the next workout. Make sure to stretch; see pages 158–59 for additional cooldown information as well as how to deal with soreness.

The Importance of Stretching and Flexibility

Whether you're a beginner to fitness or someone who's been working out for years, your flexibility is nothing to take for granted. Take a few minutes to stretch, either before or after your workout. Everyone has different strengths when it comes to how flexible particular body parts are. Below are a few stretches that you can do each and every day to help gauge and improve your overall flexibility.

A body that is too tight prevents mobility, leading to joints that seize up and can eventually lead to injury. No one wants to get sidelined by an injury, but it can happen. Simple stretches like the following help keep injuries at bay.

Forward Fold

Sitting with your legs stretched out in front of you, then reaching forward as far as possible, is a great way to test your flexibility and stretch the muscles through the back of the legs, the hamstrings, as well as muscles through your lower back. This exercise is sometimes referred to as a "sit and reach."

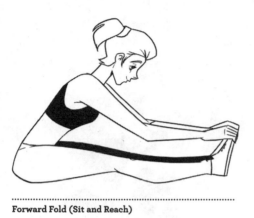

Forward Fold (Sit and Reach)

Quadriceps Stretch

Your quadriceps are located on the front of your legs above your knees. This muscle can become very tight from being sedentary, but it can also become very tight through regular strength training. It's important to maintain flexibility. Stand with a bent knee and bring your heel as close to your bottom as possible to stretch this muscle. Repeat both sides.

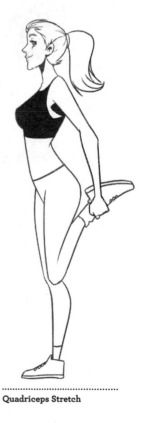

Quadriceps Stretch

Shoulder Mobility Stretch

Sitting in desks and driving in cars all day leaves our shoulders in a prone position, inhibiting flexibility. Taking a minute or two every day to open up the shoulder joint will help keep it more mobile and protected from injury. Stand with your feet hip-width apart, extend one arm up in the air, then bend your elbow bringing your hand down your back. Drop the opposite hand down, then bend the elbow bringing the fingers of each hand as close as possible. Ideally, fingertips will touch, or hands will grip one another. Repeat both sides.

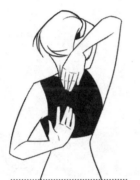

Shoulder Mobility Stretch

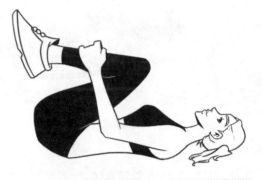

Lower Back Stretch

Lower Back Stretch

This relaxing stretch helps to take stress and tension off the lower back while helping to stretch the muscles that surround that region. Lying flat on the ground, bend both knees and pull them as close as possible into your chest. Wrap your hands around your bent legs, below the knees, squeezing them toward your chest as much as possible. Hold this stretch for at least one minute.

Side Stretch

This is a great stretch that opens up the sides of the body from the top of the ribs down to the outside of the knees. Begin by standing straight. Cross your right foot over your left foot. Extend your right arm up then over, arching your body gently to the left. Hold for thirty seconds, then repeat on the opposite side.

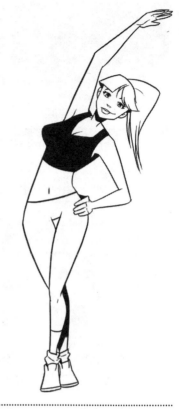

Side Stretch

WORKOUT #1

Beginner	Intermediate	Advanced
Total Workout Time		
40–45 Minutes	40–45 Minutes	50–55 Minutes
Equipment Needed: None		
Warm-Up: 10 minutes of easy cardio		

Circuit 1

(repeat 2 times; rest 1 minute between sets)	(repeat 2 times; rest 1 minute between sets)	(repeat 3 times; rest 1 minute between sets)
■ **30 Step-Ups (15 each leg)** ■ **20 Body Weight Squats** ■ **30 Donkey Kicks (15 each leg)**	■ **30 Reverse Lunge to Forward Kick (15 each leg)** ■ **40 Squat Jumps** ■ **30 Out & Ins**	■ **40 Reverse Lunge to Forward Kick (20 each leg)** ■ **60 Squat Jumps** ■ **60 Out & Ins**

Circuit 2

(repeat 2 times; rest 1 minute between sets)	(repeat 2 times; rest 1 minute between sets)	(repeat 3 times; rest 1 minute between sets)
■ **60 Jumping Jacks** ■ **30-Second Straight-Arm Plank (on knees if necessary)** ■ **60-Second Bridge**	■ **12 Burpees** ■ **45-Second Straight-Arm Plank** ■ **90-Second Bridge**	■ **18 Burpees** ■ **75-Second Straight-Arm Plank** ■ **90-Second Bridge**

Circuit 3

(repeat 2 times; rest 1 minute between sets)	(repeat 2 times; rest 1 minute between sets)	(repeat 3 times; rest 1 minute between sets)
■ **30 Lunges (15 each leg)** ■ **15 Push-Ups** ■ **30 Heel Taps**	■ **30 Lunges (15 each leg)** ■ **20 Push-Ups** ■ **60 Heel Taps**	■ **40 Lunges (20 each leg)** ■ **20 Push-Ups** ■ **90 Heel Taps**

WORKOUT #2

Beginner	Intermediate	Advanced
Total Workout Time		
35–40 Minutes	40–45 Minutes	45–50 Minutes
Equipment Needed: 1 hand-held weight between 3–10 pounds		
Warm-Up: 5 minutes of easy cardio		

Circuit 1

(1 time through; rest 2 minutes between circuits)	(1 time through; rest 2 minutes between circuits)	(1 time through; rest 2 minutes between circuits)
■ **60 Seconds Marching in Place** ■ **20 Figure-8 Shoulder Sizzlers** ■ **15 Push-Ups (on knees)** ■ **5-Minute Moderate Cardio**	■ **30 Squat Jumps** ■ **30 Figure-8 Shoulder Sizzlers** ■ **20 Plank to Push-Ups** ■ **5-Minute Moderate Cardio**	■ **40 Squat Jumps** ■ **40 Figure-8 Shoulder Sizzlers** ■ **30 Split Leg Squats (15 each leg)** ■ **30 Plank to Push-Ups** ■ **5-Minute Moderate Cardio**

Circuit 2

(1 time through; rest 2 minutes between circuits)	(1 time through; rest 2 minutes between circuits)	(1 time through; rest 2 minutes between circuits)
■ **60 Seconds Marching in Place** ■ **20 Figure-8 Shoulder Sizzlers** ■ **15 Push-Ups (on knees)** ■ **5-Minute Moderate/ Intense Cardio**	■ **30 Squat Jumps** ■ **30 Figuro 8 Shoulder Sizzlers** ■ **20 Plank to Push-Ups** ■ **5-Minute Moderate/ Intense Cardio**	■ **40 Squat Jumps** ■ **40 Figuro 8 Shoulder Sizzlers** ■ **30 Split Leg Squats (15 each leg)** ■ **30 Plank to Push-Ups** ■ **5-Minute Moderate/ Intense Cardio**

Circuit 3

(1 time through)	(1 time through)	(1 time through)
■ **60 Seconds Marching in Place** ■ **20 Figure-8 Shoulder Sizzlers** ■ **15 Push-Ups (on knees)** ■ **5-Minute Intense Cardio**	■ **30 Squat Jumps** ■ **30 Figure-8 Shoulder Sizzlers** ■ **20 Plank to Push-Ups** ■ **5-Minute Intense Cardio**	■ **40 Squat Jumps** ■ **40 Figure-8 Shoulder Sizzlers** ■ **30 Split Leg Squats (15 each leg)** ■ **30 Plank to Push-Ups** ■ **5-Minute Intense Cardio**

WORKOUT #3

Beginner	Intermediate	Advanced
	Total Workout Time	
45 Minutes	45–50 Minutes	55–60 Minutes
Equipment Needed: 1 set of hand-held weights between 5–10 pounds		
Warm-Up: 10 minutes of easy cardio		

Circuit 1

(repeat 2 times; rest 1 minute between sets)	(repeat 2 times; rest 1 minute between sets)	(repeat 3 times; rest 1 minute between sets)
▪ **30 Jumping Jacks** ▪ **30 Push-Ups (on knees)** ▪ **30 Squat to Side Kicks (15 each side)**	▪ **40 Mountain Climbers** ▪ **30 Squat Jumps** ▪ **60 Jumping Jacks**	▪ **40 Mountain Climbers** ▪ **30 Squat Jumps** ▪ **60 Jumping Jacks**

Circuit 2

(repeat 2 times; rest 1 minute between sets)	(repeat 2 times; rest 1 minute between sets)	(repeat 3 times; rest 1 minute between sets)
▪ **20 Body Weight Squats** ▪ **30 Arm Circles** ▪ **60-Second Bridge**	▪ **15 Burpees** ▪ **60-Second Straight-Arm Plank** ▪ **60-Second Bridge**	▪ **15 Burpees** ▪ **60-Second Straight-Arm Plank** ▪ **60-Second Bridge**

Circuit 3

(repeat 2 times; rest 1 minute between sets)	(repeat 2 times; rest 1 minute between sets)	(repeat 3 times; rest 1 minute between sets)
▪ **20 Lunge & Twists (10 each side)** ▪ **20 Shoulder Press Squats** ▪ **30 Heel Taps**	▪ **30 Lunge & Twists (15 each side)** ▪ **25 Shoulder Press Squats** ▪ **30-Second Side Plank (each side)**	▪ **30 Lunge & Twists (15 each side)** ▪ **25 Shoulder Press Squats** ▪ **30-Second Side Plank (each side)**

WORKOUT #4

Beginner	Intermediate	Advanced
Total Workout Time		
40–45 Minutes	45–50 Minutes	50–55 Minutes
Equipment Needed		
None	1 set of hand-held weights between 5–15 pounds	

Warm-Up: 5 minutes of easy cardio

Circuit 1

(1 time through; rest 2 minutes between circuits)	(1 time through; rest 2 minutes between circuits)	(1 time through; rest 2 minutes between circuits)
▪ 30 Body Weight Squats ▪ 30 Lunges (15 each leg) ▪ 30-Second Wall Squat ▪ 30-Second Straight-Arm Plank ▪ 2 Minutes Moderate Cardio	▪ 30 Body Weight Squats (holding weights) ▪ 30 Lunges (15 each leg; holding weights) ▪ 30-Second Wall Squat ▪ 30-Second Straight-Arm Plank ▪ 4 Minutes Moderate/ Intense Cardio	▪ 40 Body Weight Squats (holding weights) ▪ 40 Lunges (20 each leg; holding weights) ▪ 45-Second Wall Squat ▪ 45-Second Straight-Arm Plank ▪ 6 Minutes Moderate/ Intense Cardio

Circuit 2

(1 time through; rest 2 minutes between circuits)	(1 time through; rest 2 minutes between circuits)	(1 time through; rest 2 minutes between circuits)
▪ 30 Body Weight Squats ▪ 30 Lunges (15 each leg) ▪ 30-Second Wall Squat ▪ 30-Second Straight-Arm Plank ▪ 3 Minutes Moderate/ Intense Cardio	▪ 40 Body Weight Squats (holding weights) ▪ 40 Lunges (20 each leg; holding weights) ▪ 45-Second Wall Squat ▪ 45-Second Straight-Arm Plank ▪ 5 Minutes Intense Cardio	▪ 50 Body Weight Squats (holding weights) ▪ 50 Lunges (25 each leg; holding weights) ▪ 60-Second Wall Squat ▪ 60-Second Straight-Arm Plank ▪ 7 Minutes Intense Cardio

Circuit 3

(1 time through)	(1 time through)	(1 time through)
▪ 30 Body Weight Squats ▪ 30 Lunges (15 each leg) ▪ 30-Second Wall Squat ▪ 30-Second Straight-Arm Plank ▪ 4 Minutes Intense Cardio	▪ 50 Body Weight Squats (holding weights) ▪ 50 Lunges (25 each leg; holding weights) ▪ 60-Second Wall Squat ▪ 60-Second Straight-Arm Plank ▪ 6 Minutes Intense Cardio	▪ 60 Body Weight Squats (holding weights) ▪ 60 Lunges (30 each leg; holding weights) ▪ 75-Second Wall Squat ▪ 75-Second Straight Arm Plank ▪ 8 Minutes Intense Cardio

WORKOUT #5

Beginner	Intermediate	Advanced
Total Workout Time		
45–50 Minutes	45–50 Minutes	50–55 Minutes
Equipment Needed		
2 sets of hand-held weights (one heavier, one lighter) between 5–15 pounds		
Warm-Up: 5 minutes of easy cardio		

Circuit 1

Beginner	Intermediate	Advanced
(repeat 3 times; rest 1 minute between sets)	(repeat 2 times; rest 1 minute between sets)	(repeat 3 times; rest 1 minute between sets)
▪ **30 Lunges** (alternating legs; holding heavier weights)	▪ **40 Lunges (alternating legs; holding weights)**	▪ **40 Lunges (alternating legs; holding weights)**
▪ **60-Seconds High Knee Marching**	▪ **40 Jumping Jacks**	▪ **40 Jumping Jacks**
▪ **20 Abdominal Crunches**	▪ **60 Single Leg Hops (30 each foot)**	▪ **60 Single Leg Hops (30 each foot)**
	▪ **40-Second Abdominal Crunches**	▪ **40-Second Abdominal Crunches**

Circuit 2

Beginner	Intermediate	Advanced
(repeat 3 times; rest 1 minute between sets)	(repeat 2 times; rest 1 minute between sets)	(repeat 3 times; rest 1 minute between sets)
▪ **15 Shoulder Presses (heavier weights)**	▪ **20 Shoulder Presses (heavier weights)**	▪ **20 Shoulder Presses (heavier weights)**
▪ **20 Wall Push-Ups**	▪ **30 Wall Push-Ups**	▪ **30 Wall Push-Ups**
▪ **30 Step-Ups (15 each leg)**	▪ **15 Burpees**	▪ **15 Burpees**
	▪ **30 Hip Dips (15 each side)**	▪ **30 Hip Dips (15 each side)**

Circuit 3

Beginner	Intermediate	Advanced
(repeat 3 times; rest 1 minute between sets)	(repeat 2 times; rest 1 minute between sets)	(repeat 3 times; rest 1 minute between sets)
▪ **15 Lateral Arm Raises (lighter weights)**	▪ **60 Crossover Punches (lighter weights)**	▪ **60 Crossover Punches (lighter weights)**
▪ **30 Body Weight Squats**	▪ **50 Body Weight Squats**	▪ **50 Body Weight Squats**
▪ **60-Second Bridge**	▪ **40 Calf Raises**	▪ **40 Calf Raises**
	▪ **60-Second Wall Squat**	▪ **60-Second Wall Squat**

WORKOUT #6

Beginner	Intermediate	Advanced
Total Workout Time		
50–55 Minutes	45–50 Minutes	50–55 Minutes
Equipment Needed		
1 set of hand-held weights between 5–15 pounds		
Warm-Up: 10 minutes of easy cardio		

Circuit 1

Beginner	Intermediate	Advanced
(repeat 3 times; rest 1 minute between sets)	(repeat 3 times; rest 1 minute between sets)	(repeat 3 times; rest 1 minute between sets)
▪ 20 Clock Lunges (10 each side)	▪ 30 Clock Lunges (15 each side)	▪ 40 Clock Lunges (20 each side)
▪ 20 Plank & Row (maintain volume – 10 each side)	▪ 30 Plank & Row (15 each arm)	▪ 40 Plank & Row (20 each arm)
▪ 60-Second High Knee Marching	▪ 10 Broad Jumps	▪ 15 Broad Jumps

Circuit 2

Beginner	Intermediate	Advanced
(repeat 3 times; rest 1 minute between sets)	(repeat 3 times; rest 1 minute between sets)	(repeat 3 times; rest 1 minute between sets)
▪ 30 Squat to Side Kicks (15 each side)	▪ 40 Jumping Jacks	▪ 60 Jumping Jacks
▪ 10 Inchworms	▪ 15 Inchworms	▪ 20 Inchworms
▪ 30 Calf Raises	▪ 15 Plyo Jumps	▪ 25 Plyo Jumps

Circuit 3

Beginner	Intermediate	Advanced
(repeat 3 times; rest 1 minute between sets)	(repeat 3 times; rest 1 minute between sets)	(repeat 3 times; rest 1 minute between sets)
▪ 30 Donkey Kicks (15 each leg)	▪ 60-Second Back Extension	▪ 90-Second Back Extension
▪ 30-Second Back Extension	▪ 60-Second Bridge	▪ 90-Second Bridge
▪ 60-Second Bridge	▪ 30 Plank Jacks	▪ 45 Plank Jacks

WORKOUT #7

Beginner	Intermediate	Advanced
Total Workout Time		
35 Minutes	40 Minutes	40–45 Minutes
Equipment Needed: 1 set of hand-held weights between 5–15 pounds		
Warm-Up: 10 minutes of easy cardio		

Circuit 1

(repeat 3 times; rest 1 minute between sets)	(repeat 3 times; rest 1 minute between sets)	(repeat 3 times; rest 1 minute between sets)
• **30 Lunges (15 each leg; holding weights)**	• **30 Lunge & Twists (15 each side)**	• **40 Lunge & Twists (20 each side)**
• **20 Curtsy Squats (10 each leg; holding weights)**	• **30 Curtsy Squats (15 each leg; holding weights)**	• **40 Curtsy Squats (20 each leg; holding weights)**
• **30-Second High Knee Running**	• **45-Second High Knee Running**	• **60-Second High Knee Running**

Circuit 2

(repeat 3 times; rest 1 minute between sets)	(repeat 3 times; rest 1 minute between sets)	(repeat 3 times; rest 1 minute between sets)
• **15 Push-Ups (on knees if necessary)**	• **20 Push-Ups**	• **30 Push-Ups**
• **10 Tricep Dips**	• **20 Tricep Dips**	• **30 Tricep Dips**
• **30-Second Wall Squat**	• **20 Plank Jacks**	• **30 Half Burpees**

Circuit 3

(repeat 3 times; rest 1 minute between sets)	(repeat 3 times; rest 1 minute between sets)	(repeat 3 times; rest 1 minute between sets)
• **20 Plié Squats (holding weights)**	• **30 Plié Squats (holding weights)**	• **40 Plié Squats (holding weights)**
• **30-Second Plank**	• **60-Second Plank**	• **90-Second Plank**
• **20 Heel Taps**	• **10 Burpees**	• **15 Burpees**

WORKOUT #8

Beginner	Intermediate	Advanced
Total Workout Time		
45 Minutes	50 Minutes	60 Minutes
Equipment Needed		
2 sets of hand-held weights (one heavier, one lighter) between 5–15 pounds		
Warm-Up: 5-10 minutes of easy cardio		

Circuit 1

(repeat 2 times; rest 1 minute between sets)	(repeat 2 times; rest 1 minute between sets)	(repeat 2 times; rest 1 minute between sets)
• **15 Shoulder Press Squats (heavier weights)** • **20 Plank & Rows (on knees; heavier weights)** • **15 Reverse Fly (lighter weights)**	• **20 Shoulder Press Squats (heavier weights)** • **23 Plank & Rows (heavier weights)** • **20 Reverse Fly (lighter weights)**	• **25 Shoulder Press Squats (heavier weights)** • **40 Plank & Rows (heavier weights)** • **25 Reverse Fly (lighter weights)**

End Circuit 1 With:

(note: perform cardio <u>1 time</u> after completing 2 sets of Circuit 1)		(note: perform cardio <u>1 time</u> after completing 3 sets of Circuit 1)
• **2 Minutes Intense Cardio**	• **3 Minutes Intense Cardio**	• **5 Minutes Intense Cardio**

Circuit 2

(repeat 2 times; rest 1 minute between sets)	(repeat 2 times; rest 1 minute between sets)	(repeat 2 times; rest 1 minute between sets)
• **20 Lunges (10 each leg)** • **20 Plié Squats** • **20 Donkey Kicks (10 each leg)**	• **30 Lunges (15 each leg; holding heavier weights)** • **30 Plié Squats (holding heavier weights)** • **30 Donkey Kicks (15 each leg)**	• **40 Lunges (15 each leg; holding heavier weights)** • **40 Plié Squats (holding heavier weights)** • **40 Donkey Kicks (20 each leg)**

End Circuit 2 With:

(note: perform cardio <u>1 time</u> after completing 2 sets of Circuit 2)		(note: perform cardio <u>1 time</u> after completing 3 sets of Circuit 2)
• **2 Minutes Intense Cardio**	• **3 Minutes Intense Cardio**	• **5 Minutes Intense Cardio**

Circuit 3

(repeat 2 times; rest 1 minute between sets)	(repeat 2 times; rest 1 minute between sets)	(repeat 2 times; rest 1 minute between sets)
• **20 Scissor Kicks** • **20 Mountain Climbers** • **30-Second Plank**	• **30 Scissor Kicks** • **40 Mountain Climbers** • **60-Second Plank**	• **40 Scissor Kicks** • **50 Mountain Climbers** • **75-Second Plank**

End Workout With:

(note: perform cardio <u>1 time</u> after completing 2 sets of Circuit 3)		(note: perform cardio <u>1 time</u> after completing 3 sets of Circuit 3)
• **2 Minutes Intense Cardio**	• **3 Minutes Intense Cardio**	• **5 Minutes Intense Cardio**

WORKOUT #9

Beginner	Intermediate	Advanced
Total Workout Time		
40–45 Minutes	50 Minutes	55 Minutes
Equipment Needed: None		
Warm-Up: 5 minutes of easy cardio		

Circuit 1

(repeat 2 times; rest 1 minute between sets)	(repeat 2 times; rest 1 minute between sets)	(repeat 2 times; rest 1 minute between sets)
▪ **40 Jumping Jacks** ▪ **30-Second Wall Squat** ▪ **2 Minutes Moderate Cardio**	▪ **10 Burpees** ▪ **45-Second Wall Squat** ▪ **3 Minutes Moderate Cardio**	▪ **15 Burpees** ▪ **60-Second Wall Squat** ▪ **4 Minutes Moderate Cardio**

Circuit 2

(repeat 2 times; rest 1 minute between sets)	(repeat 2 times; rest 1 minute between sets)	(repeat 2 times; rest 1 minute between sets)
▪ **10 Inchworms** ▪ **30-Second Plank (on knees if necessary)** ▪ **2 Minutes Moderate/ Intense Cardio**	▪ **10 Broad Jumps** ▪ **60-Second Plank** ▪ **4 Minutes Moderate/ Intense Cardio**	▪ **15 Broad Jumps** ▪ **90-Second Plank** ▪ **5 Minutes Moderate/ Intense Cardio**

Circuit 3

(repeat 2 times; rest 1 minute between sets)	(repeat 2 times; rest 1 minute between sets)	(repeat 2 times; rest 1 minute between sets)
▪ **30 Lunges (15 each leg)** ▪ **15 Push-Ups (on knees if necessary)** ▪ **2 Minutes Intense Cardio**	▪ **40 Lunges (20 each leg)** ▪ **20 Half Burpees** ▪ **5 Minutes Intense Cardio**	▪ **50 Lunges (25 each leg)** ▪ **30 Half Burpees** ▪ **6 Minutes Intense Cardio**

WORKOUT #10

Beginner	Intermediate	Advanced
Total Workout Time		
30 Minutes	50 Minutes	55 Minutes
Equipment Needed: None		
Warm-Up:		
5–10 minutes easy cardio	5 minutes easy cardio	

Circuit 1

(Repeat easy/intense cardio combo 3 full times)	(Repeat easy/intense cardio combo 3 full times)	(Repeat easy/intense cardio combo 3 full times)
• 1 Minute Easy Cardio • 1 Minute Intense Cardio	• 1 Minute Easy Cardio • 2 Minutes Intense Cardio	• 1 Minute Easy Cardio • 3 Minutes Intense Cardio
End Circuit 1 With:		
(note: perform plank for as long as possible one time after completing Circuit 1)		
• Plank	• Plank	• Plank

Circuit 2

(Repeat high knee/rest combo 3 full times)	(Repeat burpee/rest combo 3 full times)	(Repeat burpee/rest combo 3 full times)
• 30-Second High Knee Running • 15-Second Rest	• 30-Second Burpees • 15-Second Rest	• 60-Second Burpees • 30-Second Rest
End Circuit 2 With:		
(note: perform 1 set of wall push-ups doing as many as possible after completing Circuit 2)	(note: perform 1 set of push-ups doing as many as possible after completing Circuit 2)	
• Wall Push-Ups	• Push-Ups	• Push-Ups

Circuit 3

(Repeat squat/rest combo 3 full times)	(Repeat squat/rest combo 3 full times)	(Repeat squat/rest combo 3 full times)
• 30-Second Body Weight Squats • 15-Second Rest	• 45-Second Body Weight Squats • 30-Second Rest	• 60-Second Body Weight Squats • 30-Second Rest
End Workout With:		
(note: perform 1 set of heel taps doing as many as possible after completing Circuit 3)	(note: perform 1 set of plank jacks doing as many as possible after completing Circuit 3)	
• Heel Taps	• Plank Jacks	• Plank Jacks

WORKOUT #11

Beginner	Intermediate	Advanced
Total Workout Time		
45–50 Minutes	50–55 Minutes	55–60 Minutes
Equipment Needed		
2 sets of hand-held weights (one heavier, one lighter) between 5–15 pounds		
Warm-Up: 5 minutes of easy cardio		

Circuit 1

Beginner	Intermediate	Advanced
(repeat 2 times; rest 1 minute between sets)	(repeat 2 times; rest 1 minute between sets)	(repeat 3 times; rest 1 minute between sets)
▪ **15 Shoulder Presses** (heavier weights) ▪ **15 Push-Ups** (on knees if necessary) ▪ **15 Reverse Fly** (lighter weights)	▪ **20 Shoulder Presses** (heavier weights) ▪ **20 Push-Ups** ▪ **20 Reverse Fly** (lighter weights)	▪ **20 Shoulder Presses** (heavier weights) ▪ **20 Push-Ups** ▪ **20 Reverse Fly** (lighter weights)

Circuit 2

Beginner	Intermediate	Advanced
(repeat 2 times; rest 1 minute between sets)	(repeat 2 times; rest 1 minute between sets)	(repeat 3 times; rest 1 minute between sets)
▪ **30 Body Weight Squats** ▪ **20 Clock Lunges** (10 each side) ▪ **30 Calf Raises**	▪ **50 Body Weight Squats** ▪ **30 Clock Lunges** (15 each side) ▪ **40 Calf Raises**	▪ **50 Body Weight Squats** ▪ **30 Clock Lunges** (15 each side) ▪ **40 Calf Raises**

Circuit 3

Beginner	Intermediate	Advanced
(repeat 2 times; rest 1 minute between sets)	(repeat 2 times; rest 1 minute between sets)	(repeat 3 times; rest 1 minute between sets)
▪ **14 Plank to Push-Ups** ▪ **20 Oblique Twists** (heavier weight) ▪ **30 Heel Taps**	▪ **20 Plank to Push-Ups** ▪ **30 Oblique Twists** (heavier weight) ▪ **40 Heel Taps**	▪ **20 Plank to Push-Ups** ▪ **30 Oblique Twists** (heavier weight) ▪ **40 Heel Taps**
End Workout With:		
2 minutes of easy cardio followed by 3 minutes of intense cardio	2 minutes of easy cardio followed by 5 minutes of intense cardio	2 minutes of easy cardio followed by 7 minutes of intense cardio

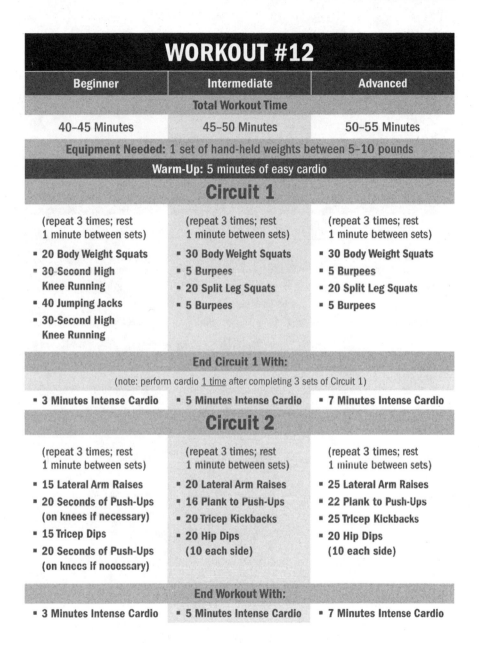

WORKOUT #12

Beginner	Intermediate	Advanced
Total Workout Time		
40–45 Minutes	45–50 Minutes	50–55 Minutes
Equipment Needed: 1 set of hand-held weights between 5–10 pounds		
Warm-Up: 5 minutes of easy cardio		

Circuit 1

(repeat 3 times; rest 1 minute between sets)	(repeat 3 times; rest 1 minute between sets)	(repeat 3 times; rest 1 minute between sets)
▪ 20 Body Weight Squats	▪ 30 Body Weight Squats	▪ 30 Body Weight Squats
▪ 30 Second High Knee Running	▪ 5 Burpees	▪ 5 Burpees
▪ 40 Jumping Jacks	▪ 20 Split Leg Squats	▪ 20 Split Leg Squats
▪ 30-Second High Knee Running	▪ 5 Burpees	▪ 5 Burpees

End Circuit 1 With:

(note: perform cardio <u>1 time</u> after completing 3 sets of Circuit 1)

▪ 3 Minutes Intense Cardio	▪ 5 Minutes Intense Cardio	▪ 7 Minutes Intense Cardio

Circuit 2

(repeat 3 times; rest 1 minute between sets)	(repeat 3 times; rest 1 minute between sets)	(repeat 3 times; rest 1 minute between sets)
▪ 15 Lateral Arm Raises	▪ 20 Lateral Arm Raises	▪ 25 Lateral Arm Raises
▪ 20 Seconds of Push-Ups (on knees if necessary)	▪ 16 Plank to Push-Ups	▪ 22 Plank to Push-Ups
▪ 15 Tricep Dips	▪ 20 Tricep Kickbacks	▪ 25 Tricep Kickbacks
▪ 20 Seconds of Push-Ups (on knees if noooissary)	▪ 20 Hip Dips (10 each side)	▪ 20 Hip Dips (10 each side)

End Workout With:

▪ 3 Minutes Intense Cardio	▪ 5 Minutes Intense Cardio	▪ 7 Minutes Intense Cardio

WORKOUT #13

Beginner	Intermediate	Advanced
Total Workout Time		
35–40 Minutes	40–45 Minutes	45–50 Minutes
Equipment Needed		
1 set of hand-held weights between 8–10 pounds	1 set of hand-held weights between 8–12 pounds	1 set of hand-held weights between 8–15 pounds

Warm-Up: 5 minutes of easy cardio

Circuit 1

(repeat 2 times; rest 1 minute between sets)	(repeat 2 times; rest 1 minute between sets)	(repeat 2 times; rest 1 minute between sets)
▪ **20 Lunges (10 each leg)** ▪ **30 Step-Ups (15 each leg)**	▪ **30 Split Leg Squats (15 each leg)** ▪ **40 Squat Jumps**	▪ **40 Split Leg Squats (20 each leg)** ▪ **60 Squat Jumps**

Circuit 2

(repeat 2 times; rest 1 minute between sets)	(repeat 2 times; rest 1 minute between sets)	(repeat 2 times; rest 1 minute between sets)
▪ **15 Shoulder Presses** ▪ **20 Crossover Punches**	▪ **20 Shoulder Presses** ▪ **35 Crossover Punches**	▪ **25 Lateral Arm Raises** ▪ **50 Crossover Punches**

Circuit 3

(repeat 2 times; rest 1 minute between sets)	(repeat 2 times; rest 1 minute between sets)	(repeat 2 times; rest 1 minute between sets)
▪ **20 Body Weight Squats** ▪ **20 Bicep Curls**	▪ **40 Body Weight Squats** ▪ **30 Bicep Curls**	▪ **60 Body Weight Squats** ▪ **40 Bicep Curls**

Circuit 4

(repeat 2 times; rest 1 minute between sets)	(repeat 2 times; rest 1 minute between sets)	(repeat 2 times; rest 1 minute between sets)
▪ **60 Jumping Jacks** ▪ **30-Second Plank**	▪ **10 Plyo Jumps** ▪ **60-Second Plank**	▪ **15 Plyo Jumps** ▪ **90-Second Plank**

End Workout With:

▪ 5 Minutes Intense Cardio	▪ 7 Minutes Intense Cardio	▪ 9 Minutes Intense Cardio

WORKOUT #14

Beginner	Intermediate	Advanced
Total Workout Time		
30 Minutes	40 Minutes	45 Minutes
Equipment Needed: None		

Warm-Up:
5 minutes of easy cardio followed by 5 minutes of moderate cardio

Circuit 1

(repeat circuit a total of 6 times; no rest in between)	(repeat circuit a total of 8 times; no rest in between)	(repeat circuit a total of 10 times; no rest in between)
▪ 1 Minute of Moderate Cardio	▪ 1 Minute of Moderate Cardio	▪ 1 Minute of Moderate Cardio
▪ 30 Seconds of Intense Cardio	▪ 45 Seconds of Intense Cardio	▪ 1 Minute of Intense Cardio
▪ 1 Minute of Easy Cardio	▪ 1 Minute of Easy Cardio	▪ 1 Minute of Easy Cardio

End Workout With:
Cool down of 5 minutes of easy cardio

WORKOUT #15

Beginner	Intermediate	Advanced
Total Workout Time		
40–45 Minutes	45–50 Minutes	50–55 Minutes
Equipment Needed		
2 sets of hand-held weights (one heavier, one lighter) between 5–15 pounds		
Warm-Up: 10 minutes of easy cardio		

Circuit 1

(repeat 3 times; rest 1 minute between sets)	(repeat 3 times; rest 1 minute between sets)	(repeat 3 times; rest 1 minute between sets)
▪ **20 Lunge & Twists (10 each side; lighter weights)**	▪ **30 Lunge & Twists (15 each side; lighter weights)**	▪ **40 Lunge & Twists (20 each side; lighter weights)**
▪ **30-Second Wall Squat**	▪ **60-Second Wall Squat**	▪ **90-Second Wall Squat**

End Circuit 1 With:

(note: perform cardio <u>1 time</u> after completing 3 sets of Circuit 1)

▪ **2 Minutes Intense Cardio**	▪ **3 Minutes Intense Cardio**	▪ **4 Minutes Intense Cardio**

Circuit 2

(repeat 3 times; rest 1 minute between sets)	(repeat 3 times; rest 1 minute between sets)	(repeat 3 times; rest 1 minute between sets)
▪ **20 Shoulder Press Squats (heavier weights)**	▪ **25 Shoulder Press Squats (heavier weights)**	▪ **30 Shoulder Press Squats (heavier weights)**
▪ **30-Second Plank**	▪ **60-Second Plank**	▪ **90-Second Plank**

End Circuit 2 With:

(note: perform cardio <u>1 time</u> after completing 3 sets of Circuit 2)

▪ **3 Minutes Intense Cardio**	▪ **4 Minutes Intense Cardio**	▪ **5 Minutes Intense Cardio**

Circuit 3

(repeat 3 times; rest 1 minute between sets)	(repeat 3 times; rest 1 minute between sets)	(repeat 3 times; rest 1 minute between sets)
▪ **20 Curtsy Squats (10 each side; holding heavier weights)**	▪ **30 Curtsy Squats (15 each side; holding heavier weights)**	▪ **40 Curtsy Squats (20 each side; holding heavier weights)**
▪ **30-Second Bridge**	▪ **60-Second Bridge**	▪ **90-Second Bridge**

End Workout With:

▪ **4 Minutes Intense Cardio**	▪ **5 Minutes Intense Cardio**	▪ **6 Minutes Intense Cardio**

WORKOUT #16

Beginner	Intermediate	Advanced
Total Workout Time		
40–45 Minutes	45–50 Minutes	50–55 Minutes
Equipment Needed		
1 set of hand-held weights between 8–10 pounds	1 set of hand-held weights between 8–12 pounds	1 set of hand-held weights between 8–15 pounds

Warm-Up: 5 minutes of easy cardio

Circuit 1

(repeat 3 times; rest 1 minute between sets)	(repeat 3 times; rest 1 minute between sets)	(repeat 3 times; rest 1 minute between sets)
• 20 Step-Ups (10 each side; holding weights) • 20 Calf Raises	• 30 Curtsy Squats (15 each side; holding weights) • 30 Calf Raises	• 40 Curtsy Squats (20 each side; holding weights) • 40 Calf Raises

End Circuit 1 With:

(note: perform cardio series <u>1 time</u> after completing 3 sets of Circuit 1)

• 1 Minute Intense Cardio • 1 Minute Easy Cardio • 1 Minute Intense Cardio	• 2 Minutes Intense Cardio • 1 Minute Easy Cardio • 2 Minutes Intense Cardio	• 3 Minutes Intense Cardio • 90 Seconds Easy Cardio • 3 Minutes Intense Cardio

Circuit 2

(repeat 3 times; rest 1 minute between sets)	(repeat 3 times; rest 1 minute between sets)	(repeat 3 times; rest 1 minute between sets)
• 10 Inchworms • 60-Second Side Plank (30 seconds each side)	• 20 Plank & Row (10 each side) • 60-Second Side Plank with 15 Hip Dips (each side)	• 30 Plank & Row (15 each side) • 60-Second Side Plank with 20 Hip Dips (each side)

End Circuit 2 With:

(note: perform cardio series <u>1 time</u> after completing 3 sets of Circuit 2)

• 1 Minute Intense Cardio • 1 Minute Easy Cardio • 1 Minute Intense Cardio	• 2 Minutes Intense Cardio • 1 Minute Easy Cardio • 2 Minutes Intense Cardio	• 3 Minutes Intense Cardio • 90 Seconds Easy Cardio • 3 Minutes Intense Cardio

Circuit 3

(repeat 3 times; rest 1 minute between sets)	(repeat 3 times; rest 1 minute between sets)	(repeat 3 times; rest 1 minute between sets)
• 30 Squat Jumps • 30-Second Back Extension	• 10 Plyo Jumps • 60-Second Back Extension	• 15 Plyo Jumps • 90-Second Back Extension

End Workout With:

• 1 Minute Intense Cardio • 1 Minute Easy Cardio • 1 Minute Intense Cardio	• 2 Minutes Intense Cardio • 1 Minute Easy Cardio • 2 Minutes Intense Cardio	• 3 Minutes Intense Cardio • 90 Seconds Easy Cardio • 3 Minutes Intense Cardio

WORKOUT #17: TABATA WORKOUT

Beginner, Intermediate and Advanced Levels

Total Workout Time: 30 Minutes

Equipment Needed: A watch or a clock

Warm-Up: 10–15 minutes of easy to moderate cardio

This workout is short, but very effective. It's appropriate for ALL THREE levels.

A Tabata workout is a set of eight 30-second intervals. Each interval is broken down into 20 seconds of hard effort work and 10 seconds of complete rest. The goal is to perform each interval completing as many exercises as possible described in the circuits below (Body Weight Squats, Push-Ups and High Knees) in 20 seconds. The intervals are performed continuously with no rest other than the 10 seconds following the seconds of hard effort work. Each circuit lasts a total of 4 minutes. Regardless of which muscles you work, there is one guarantee—you *will* feel this.

Each circuit focuses on one exercise only. You'll move from lower body strength work to upper body strength work, then finish with high-intensity cardio. Each Tabata set takes 4 minutes to complete. Pace yourself through the entire 4 minutes. It's very important to keep your eye on a clock or watch.

Circuit 1: Body Weight Squats Tabata Set

Move continuously through 8 sets of 20 seconds on/10 seconds off of body weight squats. Perform as many squats as possible in the 20 seconds, rest for 10 seconds, then go into it again. Don't stop until all 8 sets are complete. REST 2 MINUTES.

Circuit 2: Push-Ups Tabata Set
(beginner & intermediate on knees if necessary)

Move continuously through 8 sets of 20 seconds on/10 seconds off of push-ups. If you're not yet strong enough to move through the push-ups without your back hurting, rest on your knees. Perform as many push-ups as possible in the 20 seconds, rest for 10 seconds, then go into it again. Don't stop until all eight sets are complete. REST 2 MINUTES.

Circuit 3: High Knee Running Tabata Set

Move continuously through 8 sets of 20 seconds on/10 seconds off of high knee running. Perform as many high knees as possible in the 20 seconds, rest for 10 seconds, then go into it again. Don't stop until all 8 sets are complete.

WORKOUT #18

Beginner	Intermediate	Advanced
Total Workout Time		
40–45 Minutes	45–50 Minutes	45–50 Minutes
Equipment Needed		
2 sets of hand-held weights (one heavier, one lighter) between 5–15 pounds		
Warm-Up: 10 minutes of easy cardio		

Circuit 1

Beginner	Intermediate	Advanced
(repeat 2 times; rest 2 minutes between sets)	(repeat 2 times; rest 2 minutes between sets)	(repeat 2 times; rest 2 minutes between sets)
■ 40 Body Weight Squats (holding heavier weights)	■ 50 Body Weight Squats (holding heavier weights)	■ 60 Body Weight Squats (holding heavier weights)
■ 40 Lunges (20 each side; holding heavier weights)	■ 40 Lunges (20 each side; holding heavier weights)	■ 40 Lunges (20 each side; holding heavier weights)
■ 20 Crossover Punches (lighter weights)	■ 30 Crossover Punches (lighter weights)	■ 30 Crossover Punches (lighter weights)
■ 20 Push-Ups (on knees if necessary)	■ 20 Push-Ups	■ 20 Push-Ups
■ 30 High Knee Running or Marching	■ 10 Burpees	■ 15 Burpees
■ Plank (hold as long as you can)	■ Plank (hold as long as you can)	■ Plank (hold as long as you can)

Circuit 2

Beginner	Intermediate	Advanced
(repeat 2 times; rest 2 minutes between sets)	(repeat 2 times; rest 2 minutes between sets)	(repeat 2 times; rest 2 minutes between sets)
■ 50 Jumping Jacks	■ 60 Jumping Jacks	■ 70 Jumping Jacks
■ 30 Step-Ups (15 each side, holding heavier weights)	■ 40 Step-Ups (20 each side, holding heavier weights)	■ 40 Step-Ups (20 each side, holding heavier weights)
■ 30 Donkey Kicks (15 each side)	■ 30 Plank Jacks	■ 40 Plank Jacks
■ 20 Heel Taps	■ 30 Oblique Twists	■ 40 Oblique Twists
■ 20 Oblique Twists	■ 10 Broad Jumps	■ 15 Broad Jumps
■ Wall Squat (hold as long as you can)	■ Wall Squat (hold as long as you can)	■ Wall Squat (hold as long as you can)

WORKOUT #19

Beginner	Intermediate	Advanced
Total Workout Time		
40–45 Minutes	45–50 Minutes	45–50 Minutes
Equipment Needed		
2 sets of hand-held weights (one heavier, one lighter) between 5–15 pounds		
Warm-Up: 5 minutes of easy cardio		

Circuit 1

Beginner	Intermediate	Advanced
(repeat 2 times; rest 2 minutes between sets)	(repeat 2 times; rest 2 minutes between sets)	(repeat 2 times; rest 2 minutes between sets)
• **20 Lunges (10 each side)** • **30 Plié Squats (holding heavier weights)**	• **30 Split Leg Squats (15 each side; holding heavier weights)** • **40 Plié Squats (holding heavier weights)**	• **40 Split Leg Squats (20 each side; holding heavier weights)** • **50 Plié Squats (holding heavier weights)**

End Circuit 1 With:

(note: perform cardio series <u>1 time</u> after completing 2 sets of Circuit 1)

Beginner	Intermediate	Advanced
• **1 Minute Intense Cardio** • **1 Minute Easy Cardio** • **2 Minutes Intense Cardio**	• **1 Minute Intense Cardio** • **1 Minute Easy Cardio** • **3 Minutes Intense Cardio**	• **1 Minute Intense Cardio** • **1 Minute Easy Cardio** • **4 Minutes Intense Cardio**

Circuit 2

Beginner	Intermediate	Advanced
(repeat 2 times; rest 2 minutes between sets)	(repeat 2 times; rest 2 minutes between sets)	(repeat 2 times; rest 2 minutes between sets)
• **10 Shoulder Presses (heavier weights)** • **15 Lateral Arm Raises (lighter weights)**	• **15 Shoulder Presses (heavier weights)** • **20 Lateral Arm Raises (lighter weights)**	• **20 Shoulder Presses (heavier weights)** • **25 Lateral Arm Raises (lighter weights)**

End Circuit 2 With:

(note: perform cardio series <u>1 time</u> after completing 2 sets of Circuit 2)

Beginner	Intermediate	Advanced
• **1 Minute Intense Cardio** • **1 Minute Easy Cardio** • **3 Minutes Intense Cardio**	• **1 Minute Intense Cardio** • **1 Minute Easy Cardio** • **4 Minutes Intense Cardio**	• **1 Minute Intense Cardio** • **1 Minute Easy Cardio** • **5 Minutes Intense Cardio**

Circuit 3

Beginner	Intermediate	Advanced
(repeat 2 times; rest 2 minutes between sets)	(repeat 2 times; rest 2 minutes between sets)	(repeat 2 times; rest 2 minutes between sets)
• **30 Oblique Twists** • **30 Scissor Kicks** • **60-Second Plank (on knees if necessary)**	• **40 Oblique Twists** • **40 Scissor Kicks** • **90-Second Plank (on knees if necessary)**	• **50 Oblique Twists** • **60 Scissor Kicks** • **2-Minute Plank**

WORKOUT #20

Beginner	Intermediate	Advanced
Total Workout Time		
50–55 Minutes	50–55 Minutes	50–55 Minutes
Equipment Needed		
1 set of hand-held weights between 8–10 pounds	1 set of hand-held weights between 8–12 pounds	1 set of hand-held weights between 8–15 pounds

Warm-Up: 10 minutes of easy cardio

Circuit 1

(repeat 2 times; rest 2 minutes between sets)	(repeat 2 times; rest 2 minutes between sets)	(repeat 2 times; rest 2 minutes between sets)
▪ 2 Minutes Intense Cardio	▪ 2 Minutes Intense Cardio	▪ 2 Minutes Intense Cardio
▪ 20 Step-Ups (10 each leg; holding weights)	▪ 30 Step-Ups (15 each leg; holding weights)	▪ 40 Step-Ups (20 each leg; holding weights)
▪ 30 Squat Jumps	▪ 40 Squat Jumps	▪ 50 Squat Jumps
▪ 30-Second Plank	▪ 60-Second Plank	▪ 90-Second Plank

Circuit 2

(repeat 2 times; rest 2 minutes between sets)	(repeat 2 times; rest 2 minutes between sets)	(repeat 2 times; rest 2 minutes between sets)
▪ 2 Minutes Intense Cardio	▪ 2 Minutes Intense Cardio	▪ 2 Minutes Intense Cardio
▪ 30 Jumping Jacks	▪ 10 Burpees	▪ 15 Burpees
▪ 15 Push-Ups (on knees if necessary)	▪ 20 Mountain Climbers	▪ 30 Mountain Climbers
▪ 45-Second Bridge	▪ 60-Second Bridge	▪ 90-Second Bridge

Circuit 3

(repeat 2 times; rest 2 minutes between sets)	(repeat 2 times; rest 2 minutes between sets)	(repeat 2 times; rest 2 minutes between sets)
▪ 2 Minutes Intense Cardio	▪ 2 Minutes Intense Cardio	▪ 2 Minutes Intense Cardio
▪ 20 Clock Lunges	▪ 30 Clock Lunges	▪ 30 Clock Lunges
▪ 30 Body Weight Squats	▪ 40 Body Weight Squats	▪ 50 Body Weight Squats
▪ 60-Second Side Plank (30 seconds each side)	▪ 90-Second Side Plank (45 seconds each side)	▪ 2-Minute Side Plank (60 seconds each side)

WORKOUT #21

Beginner	Intermediate	Advanced
Total Workout Time		
35 Minutes	40 Minutes	45 Minutes
Equipment Needed: 1 set of hand-held weights between 5–10 pounds		
Warm-Up: 5 minutes of easy cardio		

Circuit 1

(repeat 3 times; rest 1 minute between sets)	(repeat 3 times; rest 1 minute between sets)	(repeat 3 times; rest 1 minute between sets)
• **30 Jumping Jacks**	• **40 Jumping Jacks**	• **50 Jumping Jacks**
• **20 Crossover Punches**	• **30 Crossover Punches**	• **40 Crossover Punches**
• **30-Second Plank**	• **10 Burpees**	• **15 Burpees**

Circuit 2

(repeat 3 times; rest 1 minute between sets)	(repeat 3 times; rest 1 minute between sets)	(repeat 3 times; rest 1 minute between sets)
• **30 Wall Push-Ups**	• **20 Plank to Push-Ups**	• **30 Plank to Push-Ups**
• **20 Squat Jumps**	• **40 Squat Jumps**	• **60 Squat Jumps**
• **20 Oblique Twists**	• **30 Oblique Twists**	• **40 Oblique Twists**

Circuit 3

(repeat 4 times; no rest in between)	(repeat 6 times; no rest in between)	(repeat 8 times; no rest in between)
• **30 Seconds Intense Cardio**	• **30 Seconds Intense Cardio**	• **30 Seconds Intense Cardio**
• **30 Seconds Easy Cardio**	• **30 Seconds Easy Cardio**	• **30 Seconds Easy Cardio**

WORKOUT #22

Beginner	Intermediate	Advanced
Total Workout Time		
30–35 Minutes	35–40 Minutes	40–45 Minutes
Equipment Needed		
1 set of hand-held weights between 5–10 pounds	2 sets of hand-held weights (one heavier, one lighter) between 5–15 pounds	

Warm-Up: 5 minutes of easy cardio

Circuit 1

Beginner	Intermediate	Advanced
(repeat 2 times; rest 2 minutes between sets)	(repeat 2 times; rest 2 minutes between sets)	(repeat 2 times; rest 2 minutes between sets)
▪ **15 Shoulder Press Squats**	▪ **20 Shoulder Press Squats**	▪ **25 Shoulder Press Squats**
▪ **15 Tricep Dips**	▪ **20 Tricep Dips**	▪ **25 Tricep Dips**
▪ **20 Lunge & Twists (10 each side)**	▪ **30 Lunge & Twists (15 each side; lighter weights)**	▪ **40 Lunge & Twists (20 each side; lighter weights)**
▪ **45-Second Wall Squat**	▪ **60-Second Wall Squat**	▪ **75-Second Wall Squat**

Circuit 2

Beginner	Intermediate	Advanced
(repeat 2 times; no rest between sets)	(repeat 2 times; no rest between sets)	(repeat 2 times; no rest between sets)
▪ **1 Minute Intense Cardio**	▪ **2 Minutes Intense Cardio**	▪ **3 Minute Intense Cardio**
▪ **1 Minute Easy Cardio**	▪ **1 Minute Easy Cardio**	▪ **1 Minute Easy Cardio**

Circuit 3

Beginner	Intermediate	Advanced
(repeat 2 times; rest 2 minutes between sets)	(repeat 2 times; rest 2 minutes between sets)	(repeat 2 times; rest 2 minutes between sets)
▪ **20 Wall Push-Ups**	▪ **20 Plank & Row (heavier weights)**	▪ **30 Plank & Row (heavier weights)**
▪ **20 Crossover Punches**	▪ **30 Crossover Punches (lighter weights)**	▪ **40 Crossover Punches (lighter weights)**
▪ **20 Arm Circles (holding weights)**	▪ **30 Arm Circles (holding lighter weights)**	▪ **40 Arm Circles (holding lighter weights)**
▪ **45-Second Wall Squat**	▪ **60-Second Wall Squat**	▪ **75-Second Wall Squat**

Circuit 4

Beginner	Intermediate	Advanced
(repeat 2 times; no rest between sets)	(repeat 2 times; no rest between sets)	(repeat 2 times; no rest between sets)
▪ **1 Minute Intense Cardio**	▪ **2 Minutes Intense Cardio**	▪ **3 Minutes Intense Cardio**
▪ **1 Minute Easy Cardio**	▪ **1 Minute Easy Cardio**	▪ **1 Minute Easy Cardio**

Soreness

Even the best of us experience something called delayed onset muscle soreness (DOMS). DOMS usually strikes between 18 and 24 hours after completing the last workout. Tiny microtears in our muscles are the primary reason for DOMS. As the muscles repair, we get stronger. A side effect of these microtears is soreness. Fortunately, the soreness will subside within a few days of your first workout. The best thing to do is get back to work. As tough as it might be, activity and getting the blood flowing through your muscles will help minimize ongoing soreness. DOMS is no reason to skip a workout.

Of course, stretching and drinking plenty of water will also help offset potential soreness.

Cool Down After Your Workout

If your workout has your heart rate ending on a high note, it's a good idea to take a few minutes to allow your body to cool down, letting the sweat dry off, muscles relax and heart rate drop to normal levels again. Walking at a slow-to-moderate pace and stretching using the examples on pages 133–135 are two great ways to do this. Other benefits of cooling down include:

- **Reduced Lactic Acid:** You know that burning feeling you got in your muscles as you did your burpees, shoulder presses or squats? That's from lactic acid, a substance that builds up in the muscles when we work at high intensities. Taking a nice, easy cool down can help eliminate some of the lactic acid that has accumulated.
- **Improved Flexibility:** It's normal to feel tight after a workout that uses a lot of muscles. One way to help alleviate some of the stiffness is to stretch after each workout. Stretching also helps to increase flexibility, not just in our muscles, but in our joints, too.

- **Stress Reduction:** Taking a few minutes to stretch each day is a good way to reduce stress. Muscular tension can trigger headaches and back pain. Stretching is a simple and effective way to help alleviate tense muscles associated with this type of pressure.
- **Increased Circulation:** Stretching just after a warm-up and before you start your workout is a great way to improve blood flow, increasing the amount of oxygen available to your muscles.
- **Reduced Muscle Soreness:** Stretching muscles after a workout can help to reduce the intensity of DOMS, making it easier to jump into your next workout.
- **Decreased Lower Back Pain:** Over 42 percent of working Americans report back pain as a major concern, taking a toll on the U.S. workforce at a cost of over seven billion dollars a year (1). Whether you're dealing with chronic or acute low back pain, stretching can help, and in some cases greatly diminish symptoms.

Part III:
Lasting Lifestyle Changes

"I have averaged about 1 pound a week in weight loss. More than the fact that I lost some stubborn belly fat, I am grateful for all of the information *The Belly Burn Plan* has provided me with to eat a clean diet, and why we should eat certain foods and stay away from others. For me, this definitely is the start to a better way of eating."

—DEBBIE K., AGE 55

"Thank you! I am 17 pounds lighter, no longer attached to caffeine, and just had to buy shorts two sizes smaller!"

—CHRISTINE C., AGE 38

"I'm headed for my physical this morning. I am ready to see on an 'official' scale that I have lost weight. I will happily hold my pants up (because they are too big) while standing on that scale. I can also truthfully say to the doctor that I work out three to four times a week. Ah, the winds of change create an awesome breeze!"

—KIM S., AGE 39

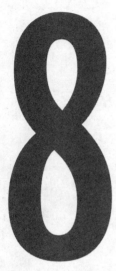

Fine Tune Your Plan:
FAQs

"Each part of *The Belly Burn Plan* was so important in helping my body in so many ways! Who knew I could eat so many good foods and lose weight while balancing everyday stress? I sleep better, move better and feel better."

—ROSEMARY W., AGE 41

As you begin *The Belly Burn Plan,* you're bound to have a question or two. Rather than try to figure it out on your own, stay on track by reviewing these frequently asked questions from Belly Burners like you who have already completed the plan. Understanding the "Why" helps us maintain motivation in the process of losing weight and getting healthier.

3-Day Cleanse

Why is the 3-Day Cleanse so low in protein?

While protein is a big component of the meal plans, it should be minimized during the 3-Day Cleanse.

Protein is a *building* macronutrient, and considered *anabolic.* We've all heard that proteins are the building blocks of muscles—and this is very true. The *building* process is usually a good thing, but if our liver, blood or kidneys are clogged or inflamed, we don't want to build on top of that. First we have to tear down, or pull out some of what's clogged up. Pathways in the liver can become congested by everyday toxins that we breathe in through the air, as well as those that are lifestyle-related, such as unhealthy foods and drinks. The 3-Day Cleanse is made of up largely *catabolic* foods, to pave the way for nutrients.

Don't worry about losing muscle! The 3-Day Cleanse is a very short phase of the program loaded with healthy foods. You'll fill your body with nutrients and rid toxins. Afterward, you'll start on Week 1 of the Meal Plan, which brings protein back into the mix.

Can I spice up the broth a bit?

The Belly Burn Broth is an important part of the 3-Day Cleanse and a healthy addition to many of the meals you'll make in the rest of *The Belly Burn Plan.* It can be an adjustment to consume something that doesn't have as much salt, and certainly not as much sugar. If you need a little extra taste in your broth, add a pinch of sea salt.

Spices are an important part of the 3-Day Cleanse. Feel free to add them liberally to everything you eat during the cleanse and throughout the remainder of *The Belly Burn Plan.* Spices possess incredible anti-inflammatory and antioxidant properties, both of which your body needs more of. Want more flavor? Try adding a couple of spices to increase the body benefits and enhance the flavor of the broth. Ginger improves circulation and digestion; curry reduces inflammation and high blood pressure; oregano fights off bacteria; and cumin suppresses the common cold and respiratory problems.

I lost a lot of weight by doing the 3-Day Cleanse. Will I continue losing weight similarly throughout the plan?

It's not uncommon to lose anywhere between 2 and 6 pounds during the 3-Day Cleanse. It's also not uncommon to gain a little bit of weight back after you complete the 3-Day Cleanse. That being said, you shouldn't gain *more* weight than you had before you began. After you begin your meal plan and workouts, you should continue seeing a slow, steady decline in weight loss throughout the entire program.

I'm getting caffeine headaches. Can I please have coffee or a diet soda?

I'll admit that caffeine, especially in coffee or tea, isn't the worst thing in the world—depending on your body type, but the whole purpose of *The Belly Burn Plan* is to get you to clean out your system and get things in working order—including fat metabolism. For many with belly fat, just one cup of coffee can throw things in reverse. In fact, caffeine has been shown to do a double whammy on our bodies by both *increasing* cortisol levels (1) and *decreasing* insulin sensitivity (2), both of which have the great potential to lead to additional fat storage.

If you're missing your daily cup of coffee, aim for organic decaffeinated coffee. If you absolutely have to have some caffeine due to withdrawal symptoms, then drink green tea. It's anti-inflammatory and contains much less caffeine than regular drip coffee.

Under no circumstances should you reach for diet soda (or any soda for that matter). Diet beverages typically contain nonnutritive sweeteners, including aspartame, sucralose (Splenda) and acesulfame potassium. Not only are these chemical ingredients toxic in your body, they also decrease insulin sensitivity. Your body gets tricked into thinking it just drank something with real sugar, so insulin comes to the rescue. Since insulin's goal, along with regulating blood sugar levels, is to store fat, drinking diet soda is the last thing you want to do—especially if you're trying to lose weight. In fact, research has shown that people who consume at least one diet soda a day are at a 67 percent increased risk of developing type 2 diabetes (3) over their lifetime.

Can I add cream to my decaffeinated coffee?

During the 3-Day Cleanse, you can add a little unsweetened almond, hemp or coconut milk, but not cow's milk. Dairy is avoided entirely through the 3-Day Cleanse. After the 3-Day Cleanse, you can add a little bit of organic cream or whole milk, if you're an Apple Type, and low-fat organic milk if you're a Pear or Inverted Pyramid Type. Hourglass Types should avoid dairy altogether until weight is under control.

Should I continue taking the probiotics and omega-3 fatty acids after the 3-Day Cleanse is over?

Yes, keep taking them daily. We're almost always lacking in an adequate amount of omega-3s and our guts can always use a good dose of healthy bacteria. Get into the habit of taking each of these supplements in the morning before you start your day. See my Recommendations on page 284.

Meal Plan

Can I eat flavored yogurt, like vanilla or strawberry?

Please avoid any flavored yogurt while doing *The Belly Burn Plan*. You'll find a Vanilla Yogurt Berry Parfait recipe on page 224, but the base of that dish is made with plain unsweetened yogurt, with a controlled amount of honey added to it. Commercially flavored varieties of yogurt, whether they're organic or not, contain a lot of unneeded sugar. Aim for plain yogurt (full-fat or low-fat, depending on your body type), which contains less *added* sugar. Keep in mind, lactose, or milk sugar, will naturally occur in all yogurts. Plain yogurt doesn't have to taste plain. You can add a lot of flavor while controlling the amount of sugar with the following ingredients:

- Berries
- Chia Seeds
- Cinnamon
- Citrus Extract
- Hemp Seeds
- Nutmeg
- Almonds
- Vanilla Extract
- Walnuts

I really want sugar or something starchy. What can I do?

It's normal to have cravings for sugar, or foods that will break down into sugar quickly, especially in the initial days after starting *The Belly Burn Plan.* With that in mind, please avoid eating sugar and refined carbs as they will quickly throw your body and all the hard work you've done in reverse. Don't cheat or start eating small amounts of anything sweet or starchy telling yourself that "it's just a little bit." This is an excuse.

Think about what the healthiest options available to you are. Low-glycemic fruit is always a good option when you really need something. Want chocolate? Have a square or two of dark chocolate. Want something salty? Eat veggies with a savory black bean dip.

Don't be surprised if you find that after a couple of weeks of going strong, you suddenly start craving the foods you've been able to go without. This is the time you need to pay attention to what's going on in your life. Stress, whether it's dealing with a sticky financial situation or the aftermath of a break up; social cues, such as going to a party with unlimited amounts of tempting food; and resting on your laurels, taking the "I've had two great weeks of eating clean and working out, therefore my body can handle a little extra food" route are all big triggers for unhealthy eating. When you feel like you might go off the rails and indulge in something you know you shouldn't, remember you're the prize at the end of the road. What's going to help you get there faster: falling back into old habits or eating clean and healthy?

Can a little slipup really slow or stall my progress?

If your slipups or cheat meals/snacks are a few times a week, then yes, you won't see the same positive progress you'd otherwise see if you hadn't cheated. If your goal is to lose weight and feel good, but you make an exception by eating candy, sugary baked goods, soda, alcohol, specialty coffee drinks, etc. on a regular basis then you're not going to see the progress you expect—even if you're working out.

If you indulge in something small, like a scoop of ice cream, a glass of wine or even a yummy homemade cookie once a week or so, your progress probably won't stall as quickly. We're all sensitive to certain foods, and since so many foods that trigger inflammation are removed in *The Belly Burn Plan,* your body will respond fairly quickly. If you reintroduce foods that are not a part of the plan, even in small amounts, and then suddenly gain weight, it's a sign that you've eaten something your body is sensitive to and it isn't serving your body to consume it.

What should I do if I slip up and eat something I shouldn't have?

Move forward. You can't undo a bad choice. We all make them from time to time, so make your next choice healthier. Don't feel guilty and don't beat yourself up over a little stumble, but try not to make it a habit. Remember, no amount of junk food can make your body feel as good as eating clean and healthy.

I have a nut allergy and can't eat nut butters. They're mentioned in the meal plan a lot. What is a good substitute?

The best substitute for any nut butter, especially for people who have nut allergies, is sunflower seed butter. When selecting a sunflower seed butter, look for a brand that doesn't contain added sugar or any partially hydrogenated oils (trans fats).

You recommend using coconut a lot. It's a saturated fat, and I'm concerned about cholesterol.

While coconut oil is a saturated fat, it contains no cholesterol. More importantly, the benefits of coconut oil—both for cooking and how it helps our bodies—are numerous.

Coconut oil is very stable. This means it won't break down when cooked or baked at high heat. The bottom line is the more stable the oil, the less the impact of free radicals on our bodies. Remember, free radicals damage our bodies much in the same way rust damages a car. The opposite is true of many common cooking oils, namely soybean, corn and canola oil.

I like to think of coconut oil as the "athlete's oil" because it gets used as energy much more efficiently than just about any other type of fat. Coconut oil is high in medium chain triglycerides, which get used up by the liver right away. This means they're much less likely to get stored as fat. Plus, coconut oil is just good for our bodies. It's antimicrobial, antibacterial and antifungal.

Why do you recommend chia seeds?

The heyday of the Chia Pet may be gone, but the benefits of chia seeds in our bodies are pretty great! Unlike flax seeds, which have to be freshly ground just before use to get the full benefit, chia seeds don't need to be ground, break down easily in our bodies and are generally more convenient. I like chia seeds because they're high in fiber (11 grams per serving) and a good source of omega-3 fatty acids. A vast majority of us lack this essential fat, so eating more chia seeds is a good way to get more of it.

There are a lot of eggs in the Meal Plan section. Is it okay if I eat egg whites instead?

I recommend that you eat the whole egg, including the yolk. The number of eggs you'll eat as part of *The Belly Burn Plan*, even if consumed daily, will not have a negative effect on your health. Of course, all bets are off if you cook your eggs in soybean, corn or canola oil—known inflammatory oils.

A number of studies in recent years have shown time and again that regular egg consumption has no impact on stroke or cardiovascular health risk (4).

What are some examples of low-glycemic fruits?

Low-glycemic fruits are always a better option than high-glycemic fruits as they'll have less of an impact on your overall blood sugar levels, helping keep hunger at bay while maintaining motivation. Here are some examples of low-glycemic fruits:

- Any berries
- Green apples
- Very hard (underripe) pears
- Grapefruit
- Cherries

What can I do with leftover nondairy milk?

Leftover nondairy milk can be used in smoothies and oatmeal.

What can I eat if I'm hungry?

The Meal Plans in *The Belly Burn Plan* all come with snack suggestions. Eat foods like these either as a morning snack or an afternoon snack. They should help keep you full until the next meal.

An important point to remember is that when you lose weight, your body requires less energy (calories) to sustain itself. A tall 180-pound active person needs more calories than a tall 150-pound active person. Your body's metabolism acts like a thermostat, holding weight steady as long as it can. As you lower the thermostat by losing weight, your body will still tell you that you need to eat more to get back to the weight at which you started. If you lose a significant amount of weight throughout *The Belly Burn Plan,* you'll eat slightly less than you did at the beginning. By that time, your body will have adjusted and you should have no problem maintaining your diet.

Each of the Belly Burn meal plans are filled with a balanced amount of nutrients that your body needs, leaving you feeling satisfied, not hungry. If you're *still* hungry, here are a few tips to get you through the day:

- *Hunger in the morning:* If you're truly hungry in the morning and not just bored, you could be lacking fat or protein, or you had too many carbs in the early a.m. hours. In that case, a tablespoon of nut butter, a handful of nuts or a hard-boiled egg should get you through until lunch.

- *Hunger in the afternoon, postlunch or predinner:* When I hear someone is both tired and hungry less than three hours after lunch, usually it tells me there is something out of whack with their blood sugar levels. Starting in the morning, make sure you're getting enough fat and protein. Too many carbs, particularly refined, can and will make you tired and hungry later in the day. All those refined carbs get converted to sugar quickly, sending your body on the infamous blood sugar roller coaster ride causing cravings.

  To get yourself back on track in the short term, drink at least twelve ounces of water. If you're still hungry after that, grab one of the snacks from your meal plan or some fresh veggies with hummus, unsalted mixed nuts, air-popped popcorn with sea salt and coconut or olive oil, a hard-boiled egg (or two), or one of the muffins from the meal plans. These foods will help you keep your blood sugar levels in check. Finding yourself hungry without a healthy snack available opens the door to poor food choices. Take the time to cut up vegetables or pop the popcorn. Have simple grab-and-go items available at all times. A handful of almonds can be a saving grace in the hour before dinner when you feel hunger setting in. Be prepared!

- *Hunger in the evening, after dinner:* A lot of people want to eat after dinner because they're bored or it has become a habit. It's really important that you try not to eat prebedtime, especially through the program. Chapter 1 goes into more detail on why, but as a recap, our bodies release human growth hormone (HGH) when we sleep, largely within the first ninety minutes. When we eat three or fewer hours before bedtime, our insulin levels tend to be more elevated than optimal. Insulin and HGH fight for rockstar position after hitting the sack. If insulin is higher, insulin always wins. Thus, HGH isn't released in the abundance in which it should be.

There is a strong chance that much of what gets eaten late at night gets stored as fat. Herbal teas, water or sparkling water are always the best bets before bedtime.

My meal plan calls for almond (or nondairy) milk. What kind should I buy?

Nondairy milks are called for in the 3-Day Cleanse because all dairy is avoided during that time frame. In lieu of nondairy milk, please buy *unsweetened* varieties of almond, rice, coconut or hemp milk. Check the ingredients label to make sure no additional sugar has been added.

Some of the recipes in my meal plan are made with applesauce. What kind should I buy?

Try to buy organic and always buy unsweetened. Applesauce without any added sugar usually states "unsweetened" on the label. Be sure to check the ingredients to make sure none is added.

I have a nut allergy and can't eat almond flour. It's added in a lot of the recipes. What is a good substitute?

Almond flour is incredibly easy to bake with and quite nutritious, too. In comparison to most baking flours, it contains no refined carbohydrates, is gluten-free, but still adds a moist, delicious flavor. If you have a nut allergy, here are a few substitutes you can use in lieu of almond flour. Keep in mind, the flavor and texture may change as you're baking with an entirely different ingredient.

ALMOND FLOUR SUBSTITUTES	
(2⅓ parts nongluten flour to 1 part starch) Use any combination	
Nongluten Flour	Starch
Oat	Arrowroot
Buckwheat	Potato
Rice	Tapioca
Garbanzo Bean	Corn (organic, non-GMO)

Do I have to follow the meal plans to a T? I find I'm spending a lot more time than usual in the kitchen.

The meal plans are guidelines to get you on track by eating the right types of foods (protein, carbs, fats) in a way that will give you energy and promote weight loss. If you don't like a particular food, then choose a substitute from the pantry staples list. The most important note is to avoid the foods that don't work for your body type.

Why do you avoid most soy products?

With the exception of fermented soy, including the gluten-free soy sauce referenced in many of the recipes, I avoid soy and don't recommend it in my practice or in any of the meal plans.

Along with soy, I don't recommend any foods that are by-products of genetically modified crops. Since over 92 percent of the soybean crops in the United States are genetically modified, I'd prefer to err on the side of caution, assuming all soy consumed will contain glyphosate, the active chemical ingredient in such crops. The focus of *The Belly Burn Plan* is to reduce or eliminated toxins in the body. While many argue that eating GMOs simply isn't bad, I can't recommend any product that has been grown to contain a synthetic chemical so potent that consumption may increase the risk of breast cancer (5) and alterations to our bodies' very own DNA (6). Unlike other legumes, by-products of soybeans are in nearly all packaged foods. In fact, it's difficult to find one processed food that doesn't contain soy. Because of the incredible prevalence of soy coupled with the avoidance of all genetically modified foods, it's not a part of *The Belly Burn Plan*.

If you're a vegetarian, there are an abundance of other substitutes that can be eaten in place of soy, including, but not limited to, a variety of other beans. You'll find a number of healthy, vegetarian-based recipes in Part IV (page 208) marked by a ⬤ icon.

What are the best anti-inflammatory foods I can eat?

Chronic inflammation tends to have a cascading effect on our health, oftentimes leading to degenerative diseases that are not reversed so easily. Remember, you're only healthy until you're not. Do what you can now to ensure you won't have to battle unneeded problems down the road.

Fortunately for you, *The Belly Burn Plan*'s diet was created with the reduction of inflammation as a priority. If you stick with the meal plan, or foods similar to it, you'll be healthier for it. I have included many of my favorite anti-inflammatory foods in *The Belly Burn Plan* recipes, such as:

- Coconut Oil
- Green Tea
- Leafy Greens
- Nuts and Seeds
- Old-Fashioned Oats
- Olive Oil
- Spices: Turmeric, Cardamom, Ginger, Garlic, Rosemary, Cloves, Cayenne Pepper, Nutmeg, Cinnamon
- Vegetables

Foods that *create* inflammation and should be avoided include:

- Alcohol (7)
- Breads and Pastas (8)
- Fried Foods (9)
- Soda, Juices (store-bought), Energy Drinks (10)
- Sugar, particularly refined (11)
- Vegetable Oils (such as corn, canola, soy) (12), (13)

Workouts and Exercises

I have no idea how to do the exercises. Help!

Take a few minutes to familiarize yourself with the exercises in Chapter 6. Most of the exercises include photo demonstrations, and all come with detailed instructions.

How hard do I have to push myself during the "intense cardio" intervals?

Hard, but to your own fitness level. An elite athlete's version of intense is very different from someone who is just starting to work out again. I like to tell people to imagine someone is chasing you . . . and you don't want to get caught. That's roughly the intensity of a hard cardio interval. It's meant to be a tough challenge, but it's incredibly rewarding.

I'm training for an endurance event and need to eat more after I finish my workout. What can I eat?

Unless you are training or working out more than ninety solid minutes, or unless your workouts are done on an empty stomach beforehand, you *do not* need to eat anything additional after you work out.

We've been conditioned to think we need sports drinks and energy bars after a workout. It's just not the case. Our livers do an amazing job storing sugar, even after a workout that's less than ninety minutes. When we eat an energy bar or drink a sports drink afterward, we're just flooding our bodies with sugar. The sugar your body doesn't need will get stored as fat. That's not to say you won't be hungry by the time your postworkout meal rolls around, but eat reasonably. There is no need to overcompensate just because you had an awesome kickboxing class.

If you are working out for more than ninety minutes, then you could use something small to eat afterward, such as a couple of hard-boiled eggs and raw vegetables or a green apple with nut butter. These provide protein for your muscles as well as the necessary carbohydrates and fat that will help keep you going until your next meal. Since the purpose of *The Belly Burn Plan* is to reduce inflammation, and most lengthy, rigorous training *increases* inflammation, please avoid bread products as a postworkout snack or meal as they trigger the inflammatory response. This means no bagels, bread, pastries, most commercial cereals, etcetera. Instead, add clean carbs with a little protein and fat. Here are a few suggestions:

- 1 apple plus 1 tablespoon almond butter and cinnamon
- ½ cup quinoa with coconut oil and raw veggies
- 1 hard-boiled egg and berries
- Whey or vegan based protein shake (see Recommendations, page 284) with chia seeds

Should I work out every day so I keep losing weight?

You really don't have to. In fact, if you've got belly fat and a lot of stress (lack of sleep, crazy work schedule, late bedtime, just a lot on your plate), then I don't recommend that you work out every day.

Your diet will help you reach your goal weight and the workouts will help you shape your body. Doing more than your body needs can actually elevate your cortisol and your adrenal response. Mentioned in Chapter 1, we already know stress affects other hormones that can make it difficult to lose weight. Don't overdo it.

I'm injured and can't work out. What should I do?

If you're injured, you need to modify your workouts. If the injury is minor, such as a strained ankle or achy knee, take pressure off those parts of your body temporarily, then ease back into your regular workouts. If the injury is more severe, such as a break or a bad sprain, take the time to allow that part of your body to heal. Depending on the location of the injury, you may be able to stay active in other ways. Use common sense and take the time you need to recover.

I'm feeling under the weather. Should I work out?

If you have a mild cold but generally feel okay, it's probably fine to work out. If you have a knock-down, drag-out illness, like the stomach flu, high fever or a severe infection, rest! It's the best thing you can do for your body. If you work out when you're too sick, you could set yourself back. Don't undo all the progress you've made. Take it easy. However, just because you feel a sniffle coming on, or you're still feeling sore from the last workout doesn't mean you should prop your feet up and call it a day. Keep moving!

I missed a workout. What do I do next?

Don't worry about it. Don't make it a habit, but sometimes life gets in the way—and that's okay. Believe it or not, when you're rushed, stressed or not feeling well, sometimes the best thing you can do for your body is get a little rest, workouts included. As soon as you're ready to start up again, pick up where you left off with the next workout.

Weight Loss

I'm losing weight, but I noticed my skin isn't as tight. Could fat be moving around?

You're born with a certain number of fat cells. Those fat cells increase and decrease in size as we gain and lose fat. Your cells stay put and don't move to a different part of your body.

Loose skin, however, happens as we get older or if there has been significant weight loss. Nearly every mother who has given birth notices that her tummy doesn't look quite the same, especially in the immediate months postpartum. The reason for this is in the connective tissue. Our connective tissue stretches and contracts with weight loss and weight gain. As we get older, our connective tissue doesn't regenerate the way it used to, so our skin gets a little looser. You can improve your skin's elasticity through lifestyle changes, including:

- **Diet:** Fresh vegetables, healthy fats and complete proteins all help to renew skin. Whether it's in the antioxidants, protein or naturally occurring collagen, a clean diet helps to restore connective tissue that helps to enhance skin's elasticity and keep circulation flowing so you always have that fresh glow.
- **Exercise:** Exercise improves your muscle tone, which gives your body a natural "lift." It also helps to push toxins out of your body via sweat.
- **Sleep:** Sleep is probably the fastest way to help your skin (we'll talk more about this in Chapter 9). We should go through five sleep cycles a night (between seven and eight hours). The first sleep cycle (in the first ninety minutes of sleep) releases the greatest amount of human growth hormone (HGH). This HGH works like the fountain of youth, helping to rebuild muscle and repair what's been broken down, including your skin.

My clothes are fitting looser, but I'm not losing weight. How is this possible?

If you notice that your clothes are fitting looser, but the scale hasn't budged, it's because you're losing body fat and gaining muscle. It's highly likely you'll start seeing the scale move soon. Until then, keep doing what you're doing because you're on the right track!

I'm not losing any weight, or I hit a plateau. Why?

Not everyone loses weight at the same pace. Some people lose weight rapidly at the beginning of *The Belly Burn Plan*, while others may only lose a couple of pounds. As long as the weight is coming off (even if only ½ pound a week), you're moving in the right direction.

If you've hit a plateau or can't lose weight, take a look at what you're eating, and ask yourself the following questions:

- Did I skip the 3-Day Cleanse?
- Am I not drinking enough water?
- Am I eating too much?
- Do I feel very full or "stuffed" after I finish eating?
- Am I snacking more than I should, even on healthy food?
- Have I been cheating on my eating plan?
- Am I still drinking caffeinated beverages?
- Am I not sleeping enough?
- Am I under a significant amount of stress?
- Am I within 5 to 10 pounds of my ideal weight?

If you answered yes to any of these questions, you could be applying the brakes to weight loss. Eating habits, caffeine, poor sleep and excess stress can all contribute to slowed weight loss.

As you get closer to your ideal weight, the needle on the scale slows as your body's internal thermostat will do what it can to hold you where you are. In this case, and assuming that you're eating healthy, focus on the workouts. Regardless of your weight, they will reignite the fire inside of you and get your metabolism moving.

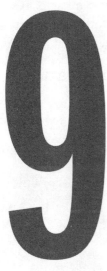

9 Sleep Your Way to a Lean Body

"My deep sleep went from about two to three hours to five-plus hours since doing *The Belly Burn Plan*. It was 100 percent due to the Plan and following the advice to stop eating three hours before bedtime."

—BECKY C., AGE 43

Jenny was having trouble finding the time to sleep. Her nonstop schedule, even on the weekends, just didn't allow it. When she finally managed to sleep, it was only for about six hours—and many of those hours were interrupted by constant tossing and turning and running through the long to-do list in her mind.

Over the past few years, Jenny noticed the bags under her eyes were more pronounced and her skin wasn't as resilient as it used to be. She knew she needed to make sleep more of a priority, but after putting the kids to bed, she wanted to spend more downtime with her husband.

The pressure Jenny put on herself to exercise still motivated her to get up early in the morning, but she didn't get the same "postworkout kick" she used to. It wasn't uncommon for Jenny to grab a coffee later in the day for a quick afternoon pick-me-up, and that was on top of her usual morning cup. Deep down, she knew that her workouts were one of the reasons she needed more sleep, but she couldn't imagine where she'd find the time to get an extra hour, even if only a couple of nights a week.

. . . .

Sleep is a simple thing, yet most of us manage to throw off this one element of health that requires little, if any, work at all. Night after night we deprive our bodies of the amount of rest needed to keep our bodies optimally healthy. Our 24/7 lifestyle leaves little room for the weary, and nonstop access to Wi-Fi means there's always work to do, email to read, candy to crush. Grocery stores, restaurants and even banks available 'round the clock all but eliminate the need to put something off for the next day. We've become conditioned to do with less sleep in the name of efficiency, even if it takes a toll on our health.

Over the past fifty years, Americans have managed to cut the average length of nightly sleep down nearly two full hours (1). In fact, 65 percent of Americans now get six or fewer hours of sleep a night (2). Shut-eye gets passed over for "doing something useful," like cleaning the house, catching up with friends or just relaxing in front of the TV. It's time to put your health first—the omission of sleep can have a cascading effect on your hormones, not to mention the amount of belly fat you collect. For the rest of the chapter, think of sleep as food. The only difference is more, not less, is better!

Most of us know that our bodies require a full seven to eight hours of sleep every night. Work and family responsibilities are usually the two most common reasons people don't get enough shut-eye. For a mother caring for an infant or young children, this is understandable and hopefully a short stage of life that eventually leads to more sleep. As a mother with three young children, I remember many sleepless nights. My kids are amazing and I love them to pieces, but they're sleep thieves, too. After baby number one, everything was great. All I had to focus on was my new little girl, and nap when she napped.

When my second little girl came along two and a half years later, I was in the throes of getting a toddler potty trained and managing the needs of a newborn. Sleep? It was a tough commodity to come by. For several months, I opted to sleep instead of staying up later to catch up with my husband, watch TV, or even do that extra load of laundry . . . and I was a lot more sane for doing so. While I worked on prioritizing my sleep, my newborn got the hang of sleeping through the night, too. Eventually, it all worked out. It's okay to prioritize your needs over household chores. The world won't fall apart and sooner or later, everything comes together.

Parenting is just one common example of how both women *and* men can get thrown off their sleep schedule. Caregivers of sick relatives, people with demanding work schedules and, well, those among us who voluntarily sacrifice sleep for social life all fall prey to less-than-stellar sleep quality. If you can identify with more than one of these types, you're not alone. The point is not to make the impossible "perfect lifetime of sleep" possible, rather to take advantage of the times you have in your life to get sleep. It's so important!

Sleep's Effect on Body Fat

A bad diet and very little activity certainly impact how much and where our bodies store fat, but the amount of sleep we get plays a vital role. Our bodies' delicate endocrine system, which regulates the hormones in our bodies, is just as dependent on sleep as it is on food and fitness. Even modest sleep deprivation over a short period of time can throw off the hormones responsible for storing more fat than our bodies need.

On a primal level, our bodies interpret sleep deprivation as a form of stress. The less we sleep, the more stressed our bodies become. This ends up affecting the amount of human growth hormone (HGH), insulin and cortisol our bodies release.

Sleep on Muscle Growth

About ninety minutes into a good night of sleep, our bodies send signals to release plenty of HGH. Not only does HGH help to repair injury to our bodies, but also to develop muscle that is broken down. This release of HGH continues to kick in about every ninety minutes and should occur about five times a night. When we don't get enough sleep, or wake often throughout the night, HGH release grinds to a halt and our bodies can't develop muscle the way that they should.

A compelling study conducted at the University of Chicago looked at two groups of people, both on a low-calorie diet, for two weeks. One group slept 5.5 hours a night, and another group slept 8.5 hours a night. That mere three-hour difference had a profound impact on each of the group members' body fat. Can you guess which group took the biggest hit? When it came to weight loss, all participants shed approximately 7 pounds of weight. Not bad, right? It turns out the group whose members slept the full 8.5 hours lost body fat, but the group whose members slept only 5.5 hours lost mostly muscle (3)!

If you regularly go to bed later than you should, or wake up too early, don't be surprised if you find it hard to develop or maintain muscle—even with a great diet or strict workout routine. Don't let the hard work you're doing to take care of your body go to waste by selling yourself short at night. Your body needs the sleep to rebuild broken-down muscle, not just to feel refreshed and alert.

Sleep on Blood Sugar Control

Insulin sensitivity is also greatly affected by sleep. Remember, it's a good thing to be sensitive to insulin. Chapter 1 told us about the relationship between insulin, insulin resistance and type 2 diabetes when it comes to the foods we eat, but it turns out that sleep plays an important role in regulating insulin as well.

When we don't get enough sleep, our cells respond much in the same way as if we ate sugar all the time—we become desensitized to insulin. When sleep is compromised—even for as little as four days—insulin sensitivity of fat cells decreases by 30 percent. Indeed, all those harmless nights of less sleep actually promote insulin resistance (4), (5). This is comparable to insulin's response between a nondiabetic and a diabetic. When fat cells don't move insulin the way they should, our body can't move the fatty acids *inside* the cell either. Fatty acids that don't get moved out of the cell increase the actual size of the cell as well as our overall body fat.

It's important to remember that we don't get rid of fat cells through diet, exercise or sleep. We simply increase and decrease the size. We now know that adequate sleep helps us move fatty acids out of the cells, shuttling them to muscles so they can be used for energy.

Sleep on Appetite

The next time you miss a couple of hours of sleep, pay attention to your appetite the following day. When we're sleep deprived for just a few days, leptin and ghrelin, two hormones that play an important role in how much we eat, are dramatically affected. When we get a good night of sleep, our bodies' level of leptin, the hormone that tells us that we're full, and our bodies' level of ghrelin, the hormone that tells us that we're hungry, are in good working order. Sleep deprivation throws these two hormones on their heads. After just two nights of less sleep, your body starts to produce less leptin (6). In other words, your body will take longer to realize that it's full. Much of the reason for this is because ghrelin levels have increased. When ghrelin increases, we think we're hungrier much more often than we really are. The result? We eat more.

While appetite isn't controlled exclusively by sleep, it plays an important role in how much we'll *want* to eat the following day. We're quick to chalk appetite up to hormones triggered by stress or premenstrual syndrome, but as you can see, that's not always the case. It's very difficult to push the plate away when your body cells are literally sending signals that you're still hungry.

Sleep on Stress

When we go to sleep, cortisol, our bodies' stress hormone, should be at its lowest point. After a full night of sleep, cortisol is topped up and we're ready to face the day, taking on any typical stressors that might come our way. When we deprive ourselves of sleep, however, cortisol levels are thrown off the next day, particularly in the evening hours when we should be winding down.

When we throw our bodies' circadian rhythm off the next day by not getting the right amount of sleep, our bodies immediately start preparing for the next night, assuming we'll want to follow the same pattern as the night before—sleep less. Shaving off a couple of hours of sleep for just one night has been shown to increase cortisol levels by 37 percent around the time you're ready to go to bed the following evening (7). This hormonal effect helps to explain why we suddenly get a second wind when it's time to turn out the lights. We might feel wiped out and incredibly tired, but falling asleep can become more difficult. Just one night's lack of sleep can actually create the same symptoms that people with insomnia experience.

Even though cortisol is attempting to give us a hand by stimulating our bodies late into the night, the day *following* a poor night of sleep, it's also rallying the troops to protect us. When we're sleep deprived, the excess cortisol produced late at night sends signals to our bodies that we're under stress, or being attacked. Remember, stress can be physical, emotional or physiological. The result of this cortisol-protected attack is extra fat storage throughout the midsection where the most protection is needed.

The best way to prevent cortisol levels from getting out of whack is by getting into the habit of going to bed at the same time every night. Burning the candle at both ends throughout the week to finish up on a work project only sets you up for a weekend of restless sleep. Similarly, staying up late at night on the weekend won't help you feel very well rested on Monday morning either. No one should avoid a social life to head home before the sun goes down all for a good night's sleep, but getting a full night of sleep lets your body reap all the benefits it deserves.

Reversing the Problem

Now comes the good news: the negative effects of sleep deprivation are completely reversible. In fact, after just a few nights of good sleep, your body starts rebounding, regulating HGH, insulin, leptin, ghrelin and cortisol back to normal levels. Your body may have a few extra pounds to lose, but rest assured that sleeping more can only *help* your body shed extra fat. Sleep is food for our brain, body and metabolism. It's just as important as a healthy meal or a vigorous workout.

Dealing with Insomnia and Sleep Loss

According to the National Sleep Foundation's 2005 poll on insomnia, approximately 50 percent of the respondents reported at least one symptom of insomnia several nights a week, and 30 percent of respondents said they dealt with symptoms of insomnia every night (8). Usually affecting more women than men, insomnia can be transient (usually the result of travel or acute illness) or chronic (common among people suffering long illness or ongoing stress).

Insomnia is characterized by the following symptoms:

- The inability to fall asleep
- Waking up frequently throughout the night
- Waking up too early
- Feeling groggy or excessively tired in the morning

Insomnia is different from the occasional night of staying up too late or waking up too early, but the long-term hormonal effects and health consequences of both are very real and happen quickly.

Getting a Good Night's Sleep

Since none of us can guarantee that we'll never have a poor night of sleep again, it's important to know what we *can* do to help keep sleepless nights at bay. More often than not, many of our day-to-day habits contribute to less-than-optimal sleep. If you're struggling with insomnia or have an occasional run-in with a sleepless night, try some of these practices to get back on track today.

- **Avoid or limit caffeine:** Too much caffeine, or drinking caffeinated beverages in general, can trigger yet another restless night of sleep. The closer to bedtime you drink caffeinated beverages, the less likely it is that you'll get a full night of sleep. The stimulation in your brain that should be tapering off a little bit is still going strong. Your best bet is to curb caffeine consumption throughout the day, but if you can't do that, don't drink anything caffeinated six or fewer hours before bedtime (9). Whenever you're feeling like you need a pick-me-up, drink a glass of water. Dehydration is subtle and can cause fatigue. Water may be just what you need. Beyond that, any type of herbal tea or sparkling water with a splash of lemon juice could hit the spot, too.

- **Go screen-free an hour before bed:** If you're in the habit of watching TV, sitting in front of your laptop or checking your phone just before lights out, you could be sending the wrong signals to your brain. Melatonin, the hormone that makes you drowsy, increases when it's dark. Late night use of tablets or handheld devices suppresses melatonin (10), keeping you up longer. Try to cut out all screens at least an hour before you go to bed. Consider reading a book or journaling before bed instead.

- **Take a relaxing bath:** Not only is a nice, long soak relaxing, it's also a great way to prep your body for bed. Just like parents do for babies, hopeful for a good night of sleep, bathing before bedtime has the same type of effect on adults. When we bathe or shower, our bodies' core temperature rises slightly. After we're out of the tub, our temperature drops, making it easier to crawl into bed for a night of rest, presumably because our bodies' temperature falls when we sleep as well (11). Sleeping at a temperature that isn't too cold and not too hot, somewhere between 60 and 68 degrees, is optimal. Temperatures below 54 and above 78 degrees have been shown to be disruptive to sleep, but somewhere between 60 and 68 degrees is the sweet spot (11).

Tonight might be a good night to turn the dial down a little on your thermostat.

- **Curb late-night eating:** When we go to sleep, our bodies' insulin levels should stay fairly low, making room for the release of HGH. When we eat too close to bedtime, our insulin levels are elevated. If they stay elevated after we go to sleep, our bodies can't rest (or digest) as well. What's more, HGH, the hormone that helps to repair our bodies, is held at bay until insulin levels fall back to normal levels. If you don't *have* to eat close to bedtime, keep in mind, it's okay to go to bed a little hungry!

- **When you've got to eat late:** If you need to eat shortly before going to bed, have a smaller meal or snack and steer clear of foods that are higher in sugar and refined carbohydrates. A bag of pretzels or bowl of ice cream might be calling your name, but if you want to sleep well, go for a piece of string cheese or handful of nuts instead. A food that's higher in protein and fat, like the cheese or nuts, will not have the same effect on your insulin levels as something more refined.

- **Sip on a cup of herbal tea:** A cup of warm, herbal tea could be just what your body needs to help wind down. Chamomile, peppermint and lemon balm teas are easy to find and do a great job relaxing the body and reducing anxiety. It's that simple. All of these teas have relaxing properties and are caffeine-free.

- **Make your "to-do" list long before bedtime:** Many people have a difficult time falling asleep because they have tomorrow's tasks on their mind, mentally ticking off all the things that have to get done when they wake up. Worrying about what you can't take care of is not only futile, but it also keeps you awake and raises anxiety levels. Avoid spending an hour staring at the ceiling when you should be sleeping by writing out a to-do list a few hours before you hit the sack. Whether it's the end of your workday or just before you prepare dinner, take five minutes to write out all those "to-dos."

- **Say no to vino:** If you regularly enjoy a glass of wine or bottle of beer at the end of the day, but wake up feeling groggy, your nightcap could be to blame. It's true that alcohol has a sedative effect on our bodies, making it easier to fall asleep. But modest alcohol consumption (one or two drinks) disrupts rapid eye movement (REM) (12). REM is the stage of sleep when we dream and store memories. Throwing off this stage of sleep not only cuts down on dreamtime, but it also affects the way we think the next day—especially when it comes to memory (13). Swap the wine for herbal tea, or water with a splash of unsweetened pomegranate juice.

- **Lights out:** Similar to the way screens can throw off our melatonin, so can regular old white light. Our brains' pineal gland, located in the center of our brains, is known as our bodies' "third eye." Even when our eyes are closed, it can sense light. When we sleep in a room that lets in too much light, our pineal gland picks up on it and significantly turns down the release of the melatonin (14). A streetlight shining through a crack in the window shade, a side lamp left on, or even an innocent night-light can throw things off. Dark curtains, turning the alarm clock away from your face and getting rid of unnecessary light when you go to bed will help you sleep through the night.

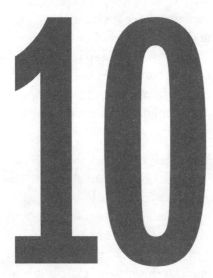

10 Prevent and Reverse Stress

"I take *The Belly Burn Plan* workouts with me to the gym, and before I know it, I'm done! If I can't make it to the gym, I choose a workout that doesn't require equipment. Some days it's hard to get started, but the minute I start a *Belly Burn* workout, I'm having fun."

—CARRIE C., AGE 41

Jenny never thought of her life as extraordinarily stressful. A little exhausting, maybe, but not stressful. That changed, however, just after the holidays when Jenny's husband was laid off from his job. He quickly found another job with a great company, but his salary took a hit. In the two months it took Jenny's husband to find new employment, the credit card bills had started mounting up. It was around that time that Jenny decided to take on more hours at work. Her additional income helped her family to maintain their standard of living and pay off debt, but also added more stress to Jenny's life.

The first few weeks of work went well. Jenny was able to get her arms around the holiday season debt and felt more financially secure. But after a while, her new routine felt harried. She was scrambling to get out of work on time to pick the kids up from school and by the time she got home, just looking at the mess made her want to cry. There just didn't seem to be enough time to do it all.

When she felt most overwhelmed, Jenny found herself eating for no good reason, and it wasn't healthy food she reached for, either. Her emotional eating usually involved dead calories from chips, cookies or the kids' school snacks. Even though it only happened once or twice a week, she'd easily add an extra five hundred to seven hundred calories in "stress food" to her diet—and that was before she prepared dinner.

· ·

Stress is a part of life that we all have to deal with. It can be real or imagined, and in many cases, based on one's perception. Regardless of what causes stress, it can have a profound and lasting impact on your overall health, including your body weight.

In a perfect world, when we encounter a stressor, like being startled by a sudden knock at the front door while watching a scary movie, stress hormones go to work pushing sugar to our muscles and narrowing the arteries to our heart, forcing blood to pump faster and harder. This is our bodies' physiological response, also called "fight or flight," that, if needed, allows our bodies to fight off a threatening enemy or run away from him. After we deal with the stressor, everything returns to normal in a relatively short period of time.

Acute stress, or dealing with a situation like this every once in a while, is something our bodies can handle. Acute stress actually has a suppressive effect on appetite. So if the stress is significant, but not long lasting, we won't necessarily reach for a bag of chips. After all, if each of us gained weight every time we encountered any sort of stress, we'd all be overweight.

Stress and Sugar

Chronic stress can take a toll on our eating habits and our weight. When we're constantly reacting to ongoing stressors, our bodies become *maladaptive* to the suppressive effect on appetite (1). It doesn't matter if the stress you're feeling is real or imagined, when you're constantly feeling anxiety over something that negatively impacts you, you'll eat more.

Stress and sugar often go hand in hand. Generally speaking, when we feel "stressed," we don't make the healthiest food choices. Candy, crackers, ice cream or soda are a few types of quick fixes that people, particularly women, tend to eat when they're dealing with a stressful situation (2). The reason for the drive toward sugary foods versus healthier foods is hardwired into our physiology. When we eat sugary comfort foods, our brains' pleasure centers turn on and release the neurotransmitter dopamine (3). Dopamine is a like the cheering section in our brains. It rewards us by making us feel good, or certainly puts us in a better mood, taking the edge off stress.

Even though scarfing down a sleeve of cookies or bowl of ice cream might ultimately leave us with regret, people with a sugar addiction tend to tune out consequences and indulge—thanks to the heavy dose of dopamine from the brain. Because that reward system is always there, ready to make us feel better, we continue to eat foods that are unhealthy. We become addicted. In fact, sugar affects our brains' receptors much in the same way alcohol and drugs do (4).

People who already have a higher waist-to-hip ratio secrete more of the hormone cortisol in response to stress than people who have leaner waistlines. Dangerous visceral fat, as opposed to the "pinchable" subcutaneous fat, occupies the abdominal region only. This makes a higher waist-to-hip ratio, like that in an Apple Type, much less healthy than in the body of someone who might weigh the same amount, but with a lower waist-to-hip-ratio, like that in a Pear Type.

Research comparing women who have more of a pronounced Apple shape over those who have more of a pronounced Pear shape shows that they simply don't manage stress as well (5). The bottom line is that stress, if not managed correctly, can have serious implications on our overall health. In some ways, too much stress can be just as bad as a terrible diet.

Emotional Eating

Since the foods we prefer in times of stress are higher in fat, more palatable and quickly metabolized, we're a lot more likely to reach for a sweet, gooey candy bar instead of a big, leafy salad. Eating these foods does nothing but pump worthless calories and lots of sugar into our bloodstream.

Though equally disastrous for either gender, women are more likely to partake in this stress-based coping mechanism (6). When we turn to food for emotional relief, we're trying to stop stress, albeit momentarily, by giving our taste buds fleeting pleasure, hence the term "comfort foods."

More often than not, when we eat in response to stress, we aren't hungry. Indeed, emotional, stress-based eating can quickly become habitual mindless eating. Mindless eating accounts for hundreds of calories that end up adding inches quickly if we don't become aware of it. Among women who eat because of stress, many overeat to the point of feeling ill. In fact, 30 percent of women say they can't stop eating "stress foods" once they start (3).

Stop Stress Eating in Its Tracks

When unhealthy eating habits take over as a means of dealing with stressful situations, the solution is to find better ways of coping. Stress-based eating is simply a bad habit, just like nail biting or teeth grinding. Eating helps buffer the stress momentarily, but it leads to a vicious cycle of guilt, more stress and weight gain.

It's worth mentioning that stress-based eating isn't the only form of indulging that can get out of hand; social and work-related eating can be just as bad. If you've ever stood next to a buffet table of tempting food at a party, or found your hand dipping into a bowl of candy on a co-worker's desk a couple of times a day, you know what I'm talking about. This type of mindless eating is a big culprit in unexpected weight gain. An extra 5 or 10 pounds of weight thanks to snacks in the office or appetizers at happy hour aren't just challenging to your mental health, but also to your joints, heart and organs.

The next time a candy bar is calling your name when a budget report is due, or a bag of chips is helping to keep conversation going between you and a few friends, consider a few of these tips to help create healthier habits, making mindless eating a thing of the past.

- **Exercise:** Just about any form of activity can help to buffer chronic stress, whether it's a quick walk around the block or a vigorous workout. When we eat chocolate or indulge in a savory snack, feel-good hormones called endorphins kick in. They're the *same* hormones that get released when we exercise. Plus, nothing beats the feeling of doing something healthy for your body.

- **Clear out the kitchen:** If it's not healthy, you don't need it. Keeping a cabinet full of your favorite snacks will only tempt you the next time you're feeling stressed. It may frustrate you at first, but in the long run, saying no to the unhealthy trigger foods and saying yes to whole, clean, nourishing foods will not only help you manage your stress, but your waistline, too!

- **Load up on nutrients:** Chances are, if you're stressed, you're lacking in vital minerals and nutrients—creating more stress. Stock your kitchen with plenty of lean proteins, such as nuts, eggs and meats; easy-to-grab vegetables and fruits, including carrots, celery, snap peas, apples and berries; and healthy fats, such as avocados and nut butters.

- **Identify your triggers:** Are you eating because it's simply time to eat and your stomach is beginning to churn, or did something just trigger you and ice cream suddenly sounds really good right now? Not only will the physical sense of hunger help cue you, so will the type of food that you're gravitating toward. Determining whether you're genuinely hungry will help you to make smarter food choices.

- **Go easy on caffeine:** Just one cup of coffee can elevate cortisol levels for hours after drinking (7). If you're already in a stressful situation, drinking any sort of caffeinated beverage could make you more irritable or anxious. Instead, downshift to significantly less or no caffeine altogether. When you first eliminate coffee, for instance, it might be easier to "step down" to green tea before switching to caffeine-free substitutes like herbal teas or Swiss water process decaffeinated coffee.

- **Keep a food journal:** Sometimes when we eat due to stress, we underestimate or forget what we consume. Making yourself accountable by writing a daily food journal, including everything—good and bad—that you've eaten can be a real eye-opener and provide incentive to not make the same mistake twice. Challenge yourself to journal your food and liquid intake for seven full days. Don't forget to write down how much water you drank, rough estimates of portion sizes and every snack you munched on. It all adds up and makes a difference, even if it's a seemingly innocuous two hundred-calorie handful of pretzels. This exercise will help you to make better choices in the present and the future.

Foods That Help You Stress Less

We already know that stress triggers cortisol to go to work, sometimes at super speed. This results in depletion of key nutrients, specifically *phosphorus*, *potassium* and *essential fatty acids*. Replenishing those nutrients will help get your body out of "fight or flight" and back to "rest and digest" faster. Here are a few incredible functional foods to eat in times of stress.

Phosphorus-rich foods: Think strong bones and teeth, muscle repair, brain function and fluid balance.

- Brazil nuts
- Cashews
- Eggs
- Halibut
- Herring
- Lentils
- Liver
- Quinoa
- Salmon
- Sunflower seeds
- Yogurt

Potassium-rich foods: Think heart and nervous system function, and fluid balance.

- Apricots
- Avocados
- Bananas
- Beets
- Cucumbers
- Dried fruit
- Lima beans
- Melons
- Sweet potatoes
- Tomatoes (all variations— raw, paste, sun-dried)

Foods containing omega-3 fatty acids: Think blood pressure regulator and inflammation fighter.

- Chia seeds
- Flax seeds, freshly ground
- Grass-fed beef
- Salmon
- Sardines
- Walnuts

Consequences of Chronic Stress on Your Body

Even if eating too much wasn't a concern, there is a strong chance that our bodies would carry extra belly fat as a result of chronic stress anyway. The cascading effect of stress hormones can pack on the pounds without eating any extra junk food at all. Our bodies have a built-in set of mechanisms called the hypothalamic-pituitary-adrenocortical (HPA) axis and the sympathoadrenal system (SAS) that help to keep hormones in good working order and balance. When these two mechanisms are overburdened with chronic stress, they become deregulated (5), leading to an unruly hormonal response.

Any time your body perceives stress, like misplacing keys five minutes before you have to be out the door for a meeting, the stress hormone, cortisol, is released. After the stressful event is over, the moment you find your keys in the refrigerator next to the milk, your cortisol levels return to normal and you carry on with your day. But let's say something happens to you each and every day that has you anxious, worried, angry or frustrated. For argument's sake, assume the stressor is an over-demanding boss at work or a baby that wakes all through the night—neither of which are particularly pleasant to deal with.

If your boss has a bad day and takes it out on you and it never happens again, or if your baby wakes once in the middle of the night, but then manages to get back to sleep, your cortisol initially rises, but then returns to normal levels fairly quickly. No harm, no foul . . . move on with your day. But if your boss is constantly on your case or if your baby hasn't slept through the night for months on end, hormones begin to respond differently. If the perceived stress is repetitive and you're not dealing with the stress appropriately, your body will respond by secreting too much cortisol. High levels of cortisol often lead to the following:

- **High blood sugar levels:** When cortisol is constantly elevated, blood sugar levels rise. Remember, our bodies are conditioned to respond to stress in a fight-or-flight manner. If we're preparing for battle, we need more energy. To get the energy, we need more sugar, thus the rise in blood sugar levels. If we don't have a real battle to fight, all the blood sugar was boosted for no good reason. When this happens, insulin acts like a "fat storage" hormone, leading to an increase in belly fat, cardiovascular disease and type 2 diabetes (8).

- **Compromised immune system:** Long-term stress can make us really sick, leading to illness, including chronic disease, by significantly diminishing the amount of protective immune cells available to our bodies (9), (10). When we experience constant stress, cortisol is constantly being released. Ironically, the helpful role of cortisol is to keep inflammation at bay. But when stress is always present, cortisol acts like a police sheriff telling his deputies, our bodies' cells, to stand down—don't fire! This leaves our bodies' immune systems unguarded and unprotected, opening the door for inflammation, viruses and infections (11).

- **Blocked nutrient absorption:** Chronic stress inhibits our bodies' ability to absorb vitamin B5, vitamin C, magnesium, zinc and potassium, creating deficiencies, low energy and decreased immunity.

- **Increased inflammation:** Too much stress quickly desensitizes our bodies to cortisol's anti-inflammatory effect (12), allowing inflammation to run rampant, triggering conditions including asthma, eczema, cardiovascular disease and other autoimmune disorders.

- **Sluggish thyroid:** Our adrenal glands, which sit on top of our kidneys, secrete all of our stress hormones, including cortisol. Excessive cortisol secretion puts our bodies in a catabolic state, meaning they're breaking down. When our bodies pick up on catabolism, they start slowing metabolism down in an effort to preserve the body, greatly affecting our thyroids.

- **Excess belly fat:** Our bodies perceive chronic stress as a threat. When our most primitive instincts take over, the goal is to hold off the threat for as long as possible by giving our bodies as much support as possible. Our bodies store fat quite efficiently around our vital organs, creating an increase in unhealthy belly fat.

The symptoms mentioned above are hallmark signs of chronic stress— all of which in some way lead to weight gain. If you have the opportunity to eliminate stress from your life, whether it's by downsizing responsibilities or letting go of people or things that pull you down, you won't regret it. To shrug off chronic stress as a badge of honor for dealing with a situation that could be better managed is playing Russian roulette with your health.

Causes of Stress and What You Can Do About Them

Before you can take control of the stress in your life, it's important to understand where it comes from. According to the American Psychological Association, the following rank as the top ten stressors (13) among adults:

1. Money
2. Work
3. Economy
4. Family Responsibilities
5. Relationships
6. Personal Health Concerns
7. Housing Costs
8. Job Stability
9. Health Problems
10. Personal Safety

Certainly, nothing can eliminate all forms of stress from our lives, but we can do our best to manage *chronic* stress. Here are some tips for how to prevent or reverse stress in your life:

- **Take 5:** Take five minutes to write down your own "top ten" list of stress makers. After you've compiled your list, take stock of what you can change to take some of the weight off your shoulders, and what you might be doing to perpetuate stress. Have you overcommitted to work or other responsibilities? Don't be afraid to seek and accept help. Are you concerned about your finances? Taking that first step to make a change can be the hardest, but once you do, you're one step closer to a solution and you'll feel that much better for it. If stress is affecting your health, not to mention your weight, all you need to do is make a few small changes to get started.

- **Say No:** It's a fantastic thing to be able to help your friends when they're in a pinch, volunteer for school events or pick up the slack on a project at work for a colleague, but don't deprioritize your own needs trying to make everyone else happy. If you have the choice, commit only to the point where you have enough free time to make you happy. Take advantage of downtime to do something for yourself, whether it's taking care of a project around the house that's been neglected or getting a massage.

- **Prioritize Your Health:** Most people think they prioritize their health, but I disagree. You know that exercise is good for you, but if you're forgoing a workout to run a few errands that could be taken care of another time, you put yourself in second place. Prioritizing *your* health means putting *you* first.

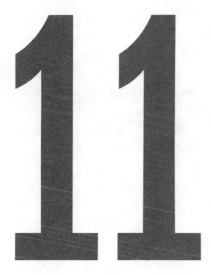

11

Track Your Progress and Stay Motivated

"*The Belly Burn Plan* delivers straightforward instruction about how to achieve results and keep going! Traci and the plan do not accept the notion that bodies have to get heavy and unhealthy with age. This plan reminded me to live life to its fullest while keeping all choices in balance with a healthy lifestyle."

—KIM T., AGE 45

Stepping on the scale was as much of a morning ritual for Jenny as getting dressed or brushing her teeth, though she knew that weighing herself every day wasn't a healthy habit. Nonetheless, her spirits were high if she lost weight, but if she gained weight, even an ounce, she was concerned, dwelling on what she had done "wrong."

After bumping into a friend who mentioned in passing that she never went on a scale because "it drove her crazy" to see her weight fluctuate, something in Jenny's mind clicked. Her friend always seemed very balanced; she didn't worry about her weight and she ate what she wanted, but in moderation. Ironically, Jenny struggled every day. Even though she tried her hardest to change her body, she saw no change. In fact, things were moving in the wrong direction entirely. Jenny wondered what it would be like if she didn't get on a scale religiously, or if she would benefit from not counting calories and cutting back on workouts. With nothing to lose, Jenny gave it a try for a week.

Instead of waking up before dawn to work out nearly every day, Jenny slept in a little more to give her body the sleep she needed. Exercise was still a priority, but she shifted her focus to shorter, high-quality workouts instead. The improvements in her sleep and workouts gave her more energy and freed up some time to think about the foods she was eating. Instead of buying foods based on what the package said, Jenny thought back to the way she ate when she felt her best. Her plate was filled with more vegetables, lean protein and healthy fat, and was virtually void of processed foods.

By the end of her weeklong healthy living trial, Jenny's pants weren't as snug and she noticed she didn't feel nearly as bloated. The greatest benefit was in her energy. She didn't feel as sluggish throughout the day and her need for coffee greatly diminished. After seven full days of sticking with this new regimen, she stepped onto the scale and saw she lost just over two pounds. Invigorated by what she saw, Jenny completely committed to her new lifestyle. Her weight continued to drop consistently—all done without counting calories or overexercising.

When it comes to tracking the progress of any diet or exercise plan that was initiated to lose weight, most of us rely on scales. If we lose weight, we're motivated to keep up the good work and if we don't lose weight . . . well, we must be doing something wrong. While knowing how much we weigh can provide a good baseline measurement, it's not always the best tool to use for gauging fitness or body composition.

Having worked with clients for nearly fifteen years, I've noticed some of the strongest people I've trained or counseled have a good 10 pounds to lose. In our culture, we're conditioned to believe that if someone is thin they're naturally healthier than their heavier counterparts. It goes without saying that being overweight is stressful on our bodies, but the real concern lies in how much body fat we have packed in between our muscles and organs. A thin person who rarely gets any activity and doesn't pay attention to diet could certainly have more body fat than someone who weighs 10 pounds more, but works out regularly and eats very clean.

There are a few key variables that will help you measure the success of *The Belly Burn Plan*. You don't need to apply all of them, but using one or two of these components will help give you a better idea of the amount of progress you're making than using a scale alone.

Measurements

Got an inch or two to lose? Measuring specific parts of your body is a great way to gauge progress, and in my opinion, a much more useful tool than the scale alone. Measuring waistline circumference is especially important; losing unneeded inches from the midsection is *always* positive and healthy. Everyone's body is different, so losing inches from other parts of the body where the fat is subcutaneous, not visceral, including the arms, chest, hips and thighs, may take a little more time for some than others.

Measuring various body parts is easy, requiring a tape measure and nothing else. Here is how to measure key areas:

- **Upper Arm:** Relax your arm and measure at the midpoint of the bicep muscle.

- **Bust:** Measure around the fullest part of your bust, over the nipple line.

- **Waist:** Wrap the measuring tape around your natural waistline, or the more narrow point.

- **Hips:** Evenly wrap the measuring tape around the widest part of your hips and buttocks.

- **Thigh:** Wrap the measuring tape around the midpoint of your thigh, in between the lowest point of your buttocks and top part of your knee.

Try to take the measurements on your bare skin, if possible (not over jeans or bulky clothing). Be as accurate as possible; don't round to the closest number. Be sure to take two measurements of each spot ensuring that you get an accurate measurement. Record and date your measurements in a notebook once every one to two weeks.

Physical Fitness

Improving your endurance or strength while losing weight is not only good for your body but it's also a great motivator. When we're able to move heavier objects or walk, jog or run faster or farther than we were able to in the past, we've almost certainly unloaded body fat and developed a little muscle. The longer we stick with it, the more the pendulum swings from higher fat and less muscle to less fat and more muscle. These measures of fitness will take your mind off the number on the scale and ensure you pay attention to the TLC you are giving parts of your body that need a little tone.

Lung Capacity

Your lung capacity, or the amount of oxygen your lungs can hold, is a strong indicator of not just your fitness, but your overall health, too. A strong lung capacity means that you're able to get more air into your lungs. The more air you get into your lungs with ease, the greater the amount of oxygen becomes available to your blood. As you work out, your muscles become a direct recipient of this oxygen, which makes working out a lot easier . . . and more comfortable.

A stronger lung capacity makes it easier to climb stairs or rush to catch a bus. Things just get easier when you can breathe easier. You don't have to wait for 10 pounds to fall off before you start noticing a difference. Your lung capacity can improve independent of your weight. Here are a couple of tests you can do each and every week that will help improve your lung capacity:

Timed Test: The timed test helps improve your cardiovascular health and your lung capacity. With the timed test, the goal is to *increase* the amount of distance you cover from the beginning to the end of the exercise.

1. Choose a cardiovascular activity (walking, running, swimming, elliptical, cycling, stair climber, rower, etc.).
2. Set a time to test yourself. I usually advise my clients to set a time between five and ten minutes.
3. Make sure to warm up for ten to fifteen minutes before starting the timed test.
4. Push yourself to see how far you can go in the amount of time you've set.

If your timed test is on a piece of cardio equipment, take note of the distance you traveled based on what the monitor reads. If your timed test is outside, take note of the point at which you started and finished.

After you complete your baseline (first) test, keep track of the distance, or make a mental note. Repeat the timed test every week to see if you can beat the distance you traveled before. Small improvements in your time by just a few seconds are a sign that you're making significant improvements to your health.

Distance Test: Similar to the timed test, the distance test is an endurance test that can help improve your cardiovascular health and increase your lung capacity. With the distance test, the goal is to *decrease* the amount of time it takes you to get from point A to point B.

1. Choose a cardiovascular activity (walking, running, swimming, elliptical, cycling, stair climber, rower, etc.).
2. Determine a distance you want to travel. I usually advise that my clients set a distance between a half mile to two miles.
3. Make sure to warm up for ten to fifteen minutes before starting the distance test.
4. Push yourself from the beginning to the end of the distance you've determined.

Record the amount of time it took you to travel the specific distance. Every week, go back and test yourself over the same distance. Did the time decrease? If so, you've gotten faster. Well done!

Body Weight Strength Tests: These tests involve using your own body weight in a way that challenges one or more groups of muscles. The goal is to measure strength. Here are a few tests you can do to measure the progress of your body's muscles:

- **Step-Ups:** As easy as it sounds, simply find a sturdy step, chair, riser or bench that is about knee height, then step up and step down, alternating legs. Complete as many step-ups as you can in sixty seconds. For further guidance, see page 126.

- **Push-Ups:** Another classic that can be done just about anywhere and anytime. Challenge yourself by completing as many push-ups as possible in sixty seconds. If you're just beginning a new fitness program, your core may not be strong enough yet. In such case, start the push-ups on your knees and graduate to holding the push-ups on your toes as your get stronger.

- **Body Weight Squats:** Body weight squats involve little more than the motion your body makes when you sit down and stand up in a chair. They're easy to do just about anywhere and work all the big muscles in your legs, hips and bottom. The goal is to complete as many squats as possible in sixty seconds. For further guidance, see page 106.

- **Wall Squat:** Similar to the body weight squats, this wall squat is the same that you'll find in the workout section of the book (see page 127). The goal with this exercise is to hold the squat as long as possible until you fatigue and can't hold yourself against the wall anymore.

With all of these tests, attempt to measure your progress once every one to two weeks. The goal is to either increase the number of repetitions you can do in sixty seconds, or increase the amount of time you can hold a wall squat.

Weighing In

I usually encourage people to weigh themselves once at the beginning of the program, then no more than once weekly (sometimes less frequently). Weighing yourself daily or even multiple times a week puts far too much pressure on you and too much value on a number.

A lot of factors can contribute to a quick increase or decrease in body weight, including hormone fluctuations, excessive sodium, the time of day weight is taken, and medications, such as birth control pills and steroids. In fact, when we first start a new exercise program, our muscles develop microtears, which can lead to temporary fluid retention due to acute inflammation. Don't worry, after the inflammation goes down and the soreness you feel after your workout goes away, so does the extra weight.

Because weight loss is unique for everyone, it's so important to use the other measurement tips to gauge your fitness and body composition. In general, if you're getting stronger during your workouts and watching the inches slowly but surely melt away, you're doing something right.

Body Mass Index versus Body Fat

Body mass index (BMI) has been used for over one hundred and fifty years as a means of determining a healthy weight based on a simple height- to-weight ratio. Commonly used by insurance companies in the United States to evaluate a variable of one's health risk, the BMI puts people in categories ranging from underweight to obese.

The formula for calculating BMI is:

$$\text{weight (lb)} \div [\text{height (in)}]^2 \times 703$$

A calculation for a person who is five-foot-four-inches weighing 140 pounds would be:

$$[140 \div (64)^2] \times 703 = 24.03$$

BMI	Weight Status
Below 18.5	Underweight
18.5 to 24.9	Normal
25.0 to 29.9	Overweight
30 or higher	Obese

According to the Centers for Disease Control and Prevention (CDC) (1), people with a BMI over the range of normal are at an increased risk of the following conditions:

- Hypertension
- Dyslipidemia (for example, high LDL cholesterol, low HDL cholesterol, or high levels of triglycerides)
- Type 2 diabetes
- Coronary heart disease
- Stroke
- Gallbladder disease
- Osteoarthritis
- Sleep apnea and respiratory problems
- Some cancers (endometrial, breast, and colon)

Active People and BMI

For health-care professionals, the BMI provides a general guideline of a healthy weight and a way to better predict the potential for disease in people twenty years of age and older. A BMI *over* 25 along with a waist circumference that is larger than normal for a person's body would indicate a potential health concern. A BMI *under* 25 and/or a normal waist circumference for a person's body may predict a person is at less of a risk of health complications.

The BMI is not a great predictor of health when it comes to people who are very active or athletic. People who are fitter tend to have more muscle mass and less fat than people who are sedentary. Because they have more muscle mass, their BMI may be greater, giving the surface impression that they're less healthy. It goes without saying that an active person with more muscle mass is healthier than a sedentary person with too much fat.

Added Benefits

In addition to the shape of your body shifting to a leaner, healthier vessel, it's highly likely you'll experience additional benefits that impact your health across the board, including the following:

Improved Sleep: One of the benefits of following *The Belly Burn Plan* is higher-quality sleep. So much of what we do throughout the day affects the way we sleep at night. By simply changing the way you eat and eliminating a few bad habits, your sleep will change for the better. Of course, you can expect to feel fatigued the night after doing one of *The Belly Burn Plan* workouts, but gradually your body will adjust to a natural rhythm of sleep.

Increased Energy: One of the big reasons many people make an effort to change their diet is because they feel unusually sluggish or lethargic throughout the day. The combination of the high-quality meal plans and recipes in *The Belly Burn Plan* along with vigorous exercise and lifestyle changes work to improve your energy levels dramatically.

Improved Immune System: When your diet is lacking vital nutrients, including minerals, vitamins and probiotics, your body's defenses are compromised. *The Belly Burn Plan* meal plans are based around whole, clean foods that give your body what it needs to stay strong and healthy. Sinus infections, achy joints and gastrointestinal distress are a few common complaints from people before starting *The Belly Burn Plan*. After completing the plan, their symptoms greatly diminish or completely disappear.

Most of us don't realize that at least 70 percent of our immune system lies within our gut. What we eat either nourishes or depletes our immunity to harmful bacteria and viruses we're exposed to every day. By eating foods that are less processed, we're building our bodies' defenses with each and every meal.

Part IV:

65 Quick and Easy Belly Burning Recipes

"The Belly Burn recipes blew me away—I can't get over how delicious every single thing tasted. And while I had to buy some ingredients that I don't normally stock, I found that I used them up because they are used in many of the recipes."

"Thank you for such a great program! It has definitely helped me make what I plan to be permanent lifestyle changes. Plus, the Sweet Potato Turkey Burgers were the best we've ever made."

The best way to control your weight is to control what you eat, and preparing your own food is the best way to do that. But let's face it, not many of us have the time to spend hours cooking in the kitchen every day. Fortunately, with *The Belly Burn Plan* you won't have to. Each of the recipes is written in an uncomplicated way using common ingredients you can find in your local grocery store. If you need some guidance finding the basic staples that are right for your body type, turn back to Chapter 4 for the list of foods that will turn your metabolism on!

There are a few ingredients in the recipes that you may not have cooked with before. Coconut oil, chia seeds and almond flour are a few great additions to keep handy in your pantry. They're all healthy and clean. More importantly, a little bit goes a long way, so they'll all last a long time!

You'll notice a few helpful icons at the beginning of each recipe that let you know whether the recipe is gluten-free, for people who don't tolerate or would like to avoid gluten in their diet; vegetarian, for people who would like to avoid meat, poultry or fish in their diet; or if the recipe freezes well, for people who want to save leftovers in the freezer for another day.

 Vegetarian   **GF** **Gluten-Free**

 Freezes Well

The purpose of *The Belly Burn Plan* is to get you to keep eating clean long after the program is over, so the recipes have to be good! Each of the recipes is full of flavor, but simple. You might even find a few recipes that quickly become comfort food in your kitchen, like the Pot Pie Crumble (page 252) or the Sweet Potato Turkey Burgers (page 262). Who says you can't put a new spin on a tried and true classic?

Belly Burn Broth

YIELD: 8 SERVINGS

This broth is packed with a cornucopia of vitamins and minerals. A staple of the 3-Day Cleanse, this broth can be made ahead and used in a number of other recipes in *The Belly Burn Plan* recipe repertoire.

- 1 gallon water
- 1 full bulb garlic, peel only outermost layer, halved
- 1 bunch cilantro
- 1 bunch parsley
- 1 bunch kale
- 1 yellow onion, halved
- 4 beets, unpeeled, halved
- 5 stalks celery, coarsely chopped
- 5 carrots, unpeeled, coarsely chopped
- 1 red potato, unpeeled, halved
- 1 cup shiitake mushrooms
- 1 cup Brussels sprouts, peel outermost layer, halved
- 1 red apple, unpeeled, seeded
- 1 teaspoon ground turmeric
- 1 teaspoon cayenne pepper
- 1 teaspoon sea salt or Himalayan crystal salt

Directions

- Add the 1 gallon of water to a large stockpot. Add all of the vegetables, herbs and the apple to the same stockpot and bring to a boil for about 20 minutes. Reduce to a simmer for about two hours.
- Allow to cool. Strain broth and discard the vegetables, herbs and fruit. Add the seasoning and serve or refrigerate in glass containers.

NUTRITION FACTS (per 1 cup serving)	
Calories	16
Fat	0g
Carbohydrate	4g
Protein	0g

3-Day Cleanse Basics

Cinnamon Berry Smoothie

YIELD: 1 SERVING

◐ ⓖⒻ

Cinnamon is a great blood sugar regulator, which helps manage hunger. This smoothie possesses the nutrients of berries, too. Simply add these ingredients to a blender, and you've got a deliciously healthy addition to your day.

- 1 cup unsweetened almond milk
- 1 cup berries (your choice, fresh or frozen)
- 1 teaspoon cinnamon
- Honey to sweeten (optional)

Directions
- Combine all of the ingredients in a blender and blend on high speed until smooth.

NUTRITION FACTS (per serving, not including honey)	
Calories	105
Fat	3g
Carbohydrate	19g
Protein	2g

Pomegranate Avocado Smoothie

YIELD: 1 SERVING

Pomegranate has been consumed for centuries . . . and for good reason. Filled with anti-inflammatory and anticancer benefits, this fruit, paired with the healthy fat of avocado, will cleanse your body from the inside out.

- 1 cup unsweetened almond milk
- ½ cup berries (any, fresh or frozen)
- ¼ cup pomegranate juice, unsweetened (see Recommendations, page 284)
- 1 tablespoon lemon juice
- ¼ avocado
- Honey to sweeten (optional)

Directions
- Combine all of the ingredients in a blender and blend on high speed until smooth.

NUTRITION FACTS (per serving, not including honey)	
Calories	216
Fat	11g
Carbohydrate	30g
Protein	1g

Basic Hummus

YIELD: 8 SERVINGS

Why buy hummus from a store when making your own is so easy? Give this recipe a try the next time you need a dip for your veggies.

- 1 can garbanzo beans (chickpeas), drained and rinsed
- ¼ cup olive oil
- 1 clove garlic, diced
- 2 tablespoons tahini (sesame paste), or unsweetened peanut butter
- Water (see directions for quantity)

- Sea salt, to taste
- **Optional add-ins:** 1 teaspoon lemon juice, ½ teaspoon cayenne pepper, ½ teaspoon adobo pepper, or ¼ cup roasted red peppers

Directions

- Combine all of the ingredients in a blender and blend on high speed until smooth. Add water gradually, starting with ½ cup until the mixture reaches your desired consistency.

NUTRITION FACTS (per serving)	
Calories	126
Fat	10g
Carbohydrate	8g
Protein	3g

Quick Tip: If you don't have tahini on hand, you can substitute unsweetened peanut butter made with no hydrogenated oils instead. A good source of calcium and iron, tahini is an ingredient you won't want to miss on your next shopping trip.

Belly Burn Cleanse Dressing

YIELD: 8 SERVINGS

This base dressing for the Pre-Cleanse is a great topper
for any salad, anytime.

- ½ cup apple cider vinegar
- ¼ cup honey
- ¼ cup olive oil
- 1 tablespoon lemon juice
- 4 cloves garlic, minced
- Dash of salt and pepper

Directions
- Whisk all of the ingredients together in a medium bowl. Store
  and refrigerate in a sealed container for up to three months.

NUTRITION FACTS (per serving)	
Calories	95
Fat	7g
Carbohydrate	9g
Protein	0g

Smoothies

Anti-Inflammatory Smoothie

YIELD: 1 SERVING

This smoothie is made with everything you need to feel great. If you've got weight you can't shake, inflammation or heat-related swelling, this will hit the spot. While all the ingredients have good anti-inflammatory properties, turmeric is one that stands out in the crowd. If turmeric isn't already a staple in your pantry, now's a good time to find this amazing spice a home.

- 1-inch piece of fresh turmeric (or ½ teaspoon ground)
- 4 strawberries (fresh or frozen)
- 1 cup spinach
- 2 tablespoons lemon juice
- 1 tablespoon honey
- 1 cup water
- 4 ice cubes

Directions
- Combine all of the ingredients in a blender and blend on high speed until smooth.

NUTRITION FACTS (per serving)	
Calories	96
Fat	0g
Carbohydrate	24g
Protein	0g

Blueberry Spinach Smoothie

YIELD: 1 SERVING

◑ GF

Spinach is an excellent source of vitamins A, C and K as well as a number of vital minerals, including iron and magnesium. This smoothie is a great way to stay hydrated, give your body a boost of energy and sneak in more than a serving of spinach, easily disguised by the more enjoyable flavor of blueberries.

- ½ cup unsweetened coconut milk
- 1 ½ cups spinach, loosely packed
- ½ cup blueberries (fresh or frozen)
- ½ tablespoon honey
- 1 teaspoon lemon juice
- ½ teaspoon cinnamon
- ½ cup water
- 3 ice cubes

Directions
- Combine all of the ingredients in a blender and blend on high speed until smooth.

NUTRITION FACTS (per serving)	
Calories	110
Fat	2g
Carbohydrate	21g
Protein	2g

Smoothies

Chia Berry Smoothie

YIELD: 1 SERVING

Chia seeds are my new favorite ingredient to cook with. A great source of omega-3 fatty acids, this energizing smoothie is full of fiber and will keep hunger at bay.

- ½ cup blueberries (fresh or frozen)
- 2 stalks celery
- 1 tablespoon chia seeds
- ½ tablespoon honey
- 4 ice cubes
- 1 cup water

Directions

- Combine all of the ingredients in a blender and blend on high speed until smooth.

NUTRITION FACTS (per serving)	
Calories	147
Fat	5g
Carbohydrate	27g
Protein	4g

Creamy Green Dream Smoothie

YIELD: 1 SERVING

This is a thick, creamy smoothie that I enjoy regularly and my kids actually love, too. Loaded with plenty of healthy fat and leafy greens, this smoothie might make a great sidekick to breakfast, lunch or even a midday snack.

- ½ avocado
- 1 cup unsweetened coconut milk
- 1 lime, juiced
- 1 cup spinach
- 1 tablespoon honey (optional)
- 2 ice cubes

Directions
- Combine all of the ingredients in a blender and blend on high speed until smooth.

NUTRITION FACTS (per serving, not including honey)	
Calories	277
Fat	16g
Carbohydrate	34g
Protein	2g

Smoothies

Green Goddess Smoothie

YIELD: 1 SERVING

Avocados aren't just for salads, and this smoothie is proof! Filled with a healthy fat that will keep hunger at bay, plenty of fiber and muscle-building protein, this smoothie makes a great meal replacement.

- ½ avocado
- 2 limes, juiced (or ¼ cup lime juice)
- 1 kiwi, peeled and halved
- 2 tablespoons vanilla protein powder (see Note)
- 1 cup water
- 1 tablespoon honey (optional)

Directions
- Combine all of the ingredients in a blender and blend on high speed until smooth.

NUTRITION FACTS (per serving, not including honey)	
Calories	366
Fat	13g
Carbohydrate	48g
Protein	19g

Note: Protein content may vary depending on the type of powder you use.

Omega Berry Smoothie

YIELD: 1 SERVING

Now's your chance to get the omega-3 fatty acids found in chia seeds. That's not all. You'll also get vitamins, fiber and a healthy dose of protein with this simple smoothie.

- 1 cup plain low-fat yogurt
- 3 tablespoons water
- ½ cup strawberries (fresh or frozen)
- ½ cup blueberries (fresh or frozen)
- 1 tablespoon chia seeds

Directions
- Combine all of the ingredients in a blender and blend on high speed until smooth.

NUTRITION FACTS (per serving)	
Calories	256
Fat	7g
Carbohydrate	36g
Protein	15g

Smoothies

Raspberry Citrus Smoothie

YIELD: 1 SERVING

Whether you enjoy this smoothie for breakfast or as a midday snack, your taste buds will love the thick, smooth texture and the tangy citrus flavor. Adding a half cup of antioxidant-powered raspberries will fuel your cells, keeping you moving all day long.

- 1 cup plain low-fat yogurt
- ½ cup raspberries (fresh or frozen)
- 1 tablespoon chia seeds
- 1 tablespoon lemon juice
- 1 teaspoon lime juice
- 1 tablespoon honey
- ½ cup water

Directions
- Combine all of the ingredients in a blender and blend on high speed until smooth.

NUTRITION FACTS (per serving)	
Calories	226
Fat	7g
Carbohydrate	38g
Protein	9g

Smoothies

Avocado Berry Smoothie

YIELD: 1 SERVING

The Belly Burn Plan keeps simple but healthy smoothies coming with this fiber-filled strawberry avocado combo.

- 1 cup strawberries (fresh or frozen)
- ½ avocado
- ½ cup unsweetened almond milk
- 2 tablespoons lemon juice
- ¼ teaspoon cinnamon
- 1 tablespoon honey
- ½ cup water

Directions
- Combine all of the ingredients in a blender and blend on high speed until smooth. If you're looking for a cool midday snack, add a few ice cubes and chill out.

NUTRITION FACTS (per serving)	
Calories	287
Fat	14g
Carbohydrate	36g
Protein	4g

Vanilla Yogurt Berry Parfait

YIELD: 1 SERVING

No matter what age you are, parfaits are fun ... and this one is healthier than most others. Take a pass on presweetened yogurts at the store and enjoy this one for breakfast or as a filling snack.

- 1 cup plain low-fat yogurt
- ½ teaspoon vanilla extract
- ½ teaspoon cinnamon
- 2 teaspoons honey
- 1 cup berries (fresh, or frozen and thawed)
- 1 tablespoon of your favorite unsalted nut

Directions

- Combine the yogurt with the vanilla, cinnamon and honey. Mix well. Layer a tall glass starting with ½ the yogurt mixture, then ½ the berries, then ½ the nuts. Repeat once more and your parfait is ready to be devoured.

NUTRITION FACTS (per serving)	
Calories	291
Fat	9g
Carbohydrate	39g
Protein	14g

Oat & Almond Breakfast Bar

YIELD: 8 SERVINGS

If you want an easy and healthy breakfast on the go, this is it. A simple spin on a traditional granola bar, these bars are light and low in sugar.

- 1 ¾ cups old-fashioned oats
- 1 teaspoon cinnamon
- 1 egg, lightly whisked
- 3 tablespoons unsweetened almond butter
- 1 banana, mashed
- 1 teaspoon vanilla extract
- ½ cup water

Directions
- Preheat the oven to 350°F. Lightly grease or line an 8x8-inch pan with parchment paper.
- In a medium bowl, mix together the oats and cinnamon.
- In a smaller bowl, combine the egg, almond butter, banana and vanilla. After the egg mixture is thoroughly blended, add to oats and cinnamon. Finally, add the water. Continue stirring mixture until water is thoroughly absorbed (about 30 seconds).
- Pour the mixture in the prepared pan. Bake for 25 minutes, or until edges become lightly browned. Allow to cool before serving.

NUTRITION FACTS (per serving)	
Calories	117
Fat	5g
Carbohydrate	15g
Protein	4g

Breakfasts

Overnight Chia Seed Oatmeal

YIELD: 1 SERVING

Getting the nutrients you need to start your day doesn't need to take much time. Full of fiber and omega-3 fatty acids, these overnight oats are a powerhouse of a breakfast, providing sustained energy all morning long.

- ⅓ cup old-fashioned oats
- 2 tablespoons chia seeds
- 1 tablespoon honey
- ½ teaspoon cinnamon
- ½ teaspoon vanilla extract
- ¼ teaspoon lemon juice
- ¾ cup water

Directions
- Combine all of the ingredients in a mason jar or sealable container. Shake vigorously and refrigerate overnight.

NUTRITION FACTS (per serving)	
Calories	284
Fat	10g
Carbohydrate	45g
Protein	9g

Quick Tip: Just one serving of chia seeds, two tablespoons, is filled with 11 grams of fiber. Plus, you'll get a healthy dose of magnesium, calcium, iron and omega-3 fatty acids. Add to oatmeal or smoothies for an extra shot of nutrition.

Banana Cinnamon Muffins

YIELD: 12 MUFFINS

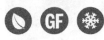

The next time you're craving something warm and sweet for breakfast, but don't want to deal with the guilt, try this grain-free, low-sugar version of a traditional bakery classic.

- 3 ½ cups almond flour
- 3 teaspoons cinnamon
- 2 teaspoons baking soda
- 6 bananas, mashed
- 4 eggs, lightly beaten
- 2 teaspoon vanilla extract
- 1 ½ to 2 cups almond milk, unsweetened

Directions
- Preheat the oven to 350°F. Line a muffin tin with paper cups, or lightly grease with coconut oil.
- In a large bowl, add the almond flour, cinnamon and baking soda. Mix well and set aside.
- In a medium bowl, combine the mashed bananas, eggs and vanilla.
- Once the banana mixture is well-mixed, add to the almond base and mix until grainy. Slowly add the milk, ¼ cup at a time. The consistency should be slightly thicker than pancake batter.
- Pour the mixture into the baking cups, about ⅔ full. Bake for 22 to 25 minutes, or until tops are golden brown. And voilà!

NUTRITION FACTS (per serving)	
Calories	190
Fat	12g
Carbohydrate	18g
Protein	4g

Breakfasts

Chocolate Coconut Energy Muffins

YIELD: 12 MUFFINS

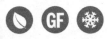

Give your metabolism a boost with this chocolate-coconut combo.

- 1 cup plus 1 tablespoon oat flour
- 1 cup plus 1 tablespoon almond flour
- ½ cup shredded coconut
- ½ cup unsweetened cocoa powder
- 1 teaspoon baking soda
- ¾ cup coconut oil, melted
- ½ cup plus 1 tablespoon applesauce
- ⅓ cup honey
- 1 teaspoon vanilla extract

Directions
- Preheat the oven to 350°F. Line a muffin tin with paper cups, or lightly grease with coconut oil.
- Combine the flours, shredded coconut, cocoa powder and baking soda in a large bowl. Mix until thoroughly combined.
- In a small bowl, combine coconut oil, applesauce, honey and vanilla. Whisk until well-blended.
- Pour wet ingredients into the flour mixture. Mix thoroughly. Ladle the chocolate mixture into the muffin cups, about ⅔ full. Bake on the top rack for 19 to 22 minutes. This muffin recipe does not rise quite as high as other muffins; be careful not to overcook.

NUTRITION FACTS (per serving)	
Calories	213
Fat	14g
Carbohydrate	22g
Protein	3g

Lemon Chia Seed Muffins

YIELD: 12 MUFFINS

This lemony muffin makes a great addition to a healthy breakfast. Or enjoy it as a snack any time of the day.

- 2 cups almond flour
- 2 teaspoons baking powder
- ¼ cup honey
- ¼ cup unsweetened almond milk
- 2 tablespoons lemon juice
- 1 teaspoon vanilla extract
- Zest of 1 lemon
- 3 eggs, room temperature and lightly whisked
- ¼ cup chia seeds

Directions

- Preheat the oven to 350°F. Line a muffin tin with paper cups, or lightly grease with coconut oil.
- In a medium bowl, combine the almond flour and baking powder. Mix well.
- In a smaller bowl, combine the honey, almond milk, lemon juice, vanilla and lemon zest. After the mixture is combined, add to the almond flour mixture and combine thoroughly.
- Slowly fold in the eggs followed by the chia seeds. After the chia seeds look evenly distributed, pour the mixture into the muffin cups, about ⅔ full. Bake for 20 minutes, or until muffins are no longer soft in the middle. Allow to cool before serving.

NUTRITION FACTS (per serving)	
Calories	169
Fat	12g
Carbohydrate	12g
Protein	4g

Breakfasts

Double Chocolate Protein Muffins

YIELD: 12 MUFFINS

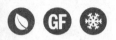

Not to be mistaken for chocolate cake, this sweet, moist, super-chocolaty muffin will not only satisfy your craving for cocoa, but give you sustained energy, in part thanks to the medium chain triglycerides from the coconut oil.

- 1 ½ cups oat flour
- ½ cup chocolate protein powder
- ⅜ cup unsweetened cocoa powder
- ¾ teaspoon baking soda
- 3 eggs, lightly whisked
- ⅜ cup coconut oil
- 4 ½ tablespoons honey
- ¾ teaspoon vanilla extract
- ¾ cup unsweetened almond milk plus 2 tablespoons reserved

Directions

- Preheat the oven to 400°F. Line a muffin tin with paper cups, or lightly grease with coconut oil.
- Combine the oat flour, protein powder, cocoa powder and baking soda in a medium-size bowl. Mix well and set aside.
- In a small bowl, mix together the eggs, coconut oil, honey and vanilla. Add the egg mixture to the dry ingredients, blending completely. Slowly add in the almond milk. The consistency of the muffin batter should be *pourable*, not scoopable. Continue adding until you get the appropriate consistency. Add 2 additional tablespoons of almond milk, if necessary.
- Pour the batter into the muffin cups, about ⅔ full. Bake for 15 to 17 minutes, or until muffins pass the toothpick test. Allow to cool before serving.

NUTRITION FACTS (per serving)	
Calories (per serving)	196
Fat	10g
Carbohydrate	19g
Protein	8g

Quick Tip: You can make oat flour from old-fashioned oats. Simply grind them up in a clean coffee grinder and in about two minutes, you'll end up with oat flour.

Quinoa Protein Power Muffins

YIELD: 12 MUFFINS

A nice balance of protein, carbohydrate and fat, these Quinoa Power Muffins make for part of a healthy breakfast or midday snack.

- ½ cup quinoa
- 1 cup water
- ½ cup unsweetened almond butter
- ¼ cup honey
- 1 teaspoon vanilla
- 3 eggs, lightly whisked
- 1 cup oats
- ½ teaspoon baking soda
- ½ teaspoon baking powder

Directions

- Preheat the oven to 350°F. Line a muffin tin with baking cups, or lightly grease with coconut oil.
- In a medium saucepan, combine the quinoa and water. Bring to a boil, then reduce heat to a simmer. Cover and cook until the quinoa has absorbed all of the liquid, about 18 to 20 minutes. Remove from heat and place in refrigerator until it is warm to the touch.
- In a large mixing bowl, combine the almond butter, honey and vanilla. Mix thoroughly. Add in the eggs and continue mixing until the mixture is smooth. Stir in the oats and cooked quinoa. Lastly, add in the baking soda and baking powder.
- Ladle the mixture into the muffin cups, about ⅔ full. Bake for 16 to 18 minutes, or until tops of muffins begin to brown. Allow to cool before serving.

NUTRITION FACTS (per serving)	
Calories	156
Fat	7g
Carbohydrate	23g
Protein	4g

Strawberry Muffins

YIELD: 12 MUFFINS

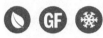

Strawberries make just about anything taste good, including muffins. This freezer-friendly recipe means you save time later in the week when you're looking for a midafternoon snack.

- 1 ½ cups oat flour
- 1 ½ cups almond flour
- ¾ teaspoon cinnamon
- ½ teaspoon ground nutmeg
- 1 ½ teaspoons baking soda
- 4 eggs, lightly whisked
- 4 ½ tablespoons honey
- ⅓ cup coconut milk, unsweetened
- 1 ½ teaspoons vanilla extract
- 1 ½ cups strawberries (fresh), chopped

Directions

- Preheat the oven to 400°F. Line a muffin tin with baking cups, or lightly grease with coconut oil. Set aside.
- Combine all of the flours, cinnamon, nutmeg and baking soda in a medium bowl. In a small bowl, combine the eggs, honey, coconut milk and vanilla. Mix thoroughly.
- Add the wet ingredients to the dry ingredients until blended. Finally, gently fold in the strawberries. Be careful not to overfold and break apart the berries.
- Pour the mixture into the baking cups, about ⅔ full. Bake for 13 to 15 minutes, or until tops are golden brown. Allow to cool before serving.

NUTRITION FACTS (per serving)	
Calories	197
Fat	10g
Carbohydrate	19g
Protein	8g

Salads & Dressings

Black Bean & Tomato Salad

YIELD: 4 SERVINGS

Make this simple salad for a side dish, a satisfying dinner or as a tasty snack. Full of nutrients, including detoxifying cilantro and nourishing olive oil, this black bean and tomato salad will fill you up while giving your body the vitamins and minerals it needs.

- 1 can black beans, drained and rinsed
- 1 cup diced tomatoes
- 3 scallions, chopped
- ¼ cup cilantro, coarsely chopped
- 2 limes, juiced
- 3 tablespoons olive oil
- ¼ teaspoon sea salt

Directions
- Combine all of the ingredients in a medium bowl. Toss gently, chill and enjoy.

NUTRITION FACTS (per serving)	
Calories	204
Fat	11g
Carbohydrate	20g
Protein	7g

Quick Tip: Look for BPA-free cans. Aluminum cans that have a plastic lining on the inside contain Bisphenol A, a chemical compound associated with health concerns, increasing the risk of birth defects, behavioral problems and raising the risk of obesity. Most companies selling products in BPA-free cans state so right on the label.

Broccoli Jicama Detox Salad

YIELD: 8 SERVINGS

Jicama and broccoli make a fantastic salad duo. Full of fiber, flavor and lots of crunch, this dish can be made ahead and enjoyed all week long.

Salad
- 4 cups broccoli, chopped into small florets
- 3 ½ cups jicama, chopped into small pieces
- 3 cups red cabbage, chopped
- 1 cup diced yellow onions
- 3 cloves garlic, pressed or minced

Dressing
- ½ cup fresh orange juice (from 1 orange)
- ⅓ cup balsamic vinegar
- ¼ cup olive oil
- 1 tablespoon honey
- Dash of sea salt

Directions
- Place all of the vegetables in a large mixing bowl and set aside. In a small bowl, combine all of the dressing ingredients and whisk thoroughly.
- Add the dressing to the vegetable mixture and toss to coat. Serve immediately or if you prefer, chill before serving.

NUTRITION FACTS (per serving)	
Calories	150
Fat	6g
Carbohydrate	21g
Protein	3g

Chickpea & Tomato Salad

YIELD: 6 SERVINGS

Take a break from your caprese salad, and give this cheese-free chickpea salad a try instead. Make for a light lunch or serve as a healthy side for dinner.

- 1 can garbanzo beans (chickpeas), drained and rinsed
- 1 pint cherry tomatoes, halved
- 1 cup chopped yellow onions
- 2 tablespoons olive oil
- 2 tablespoons balsamic vinegar
- ½ teaspoon sea salt
- ½ teaspoon pepper
- ½ cup fresh basil, chiffonade (see Note)

Directions
- Combine the garbanzo beans, tomatoes and onions in a large bowl.
- In a small bowl, whisk together the olive oil, vinegar, sea salt and pepper to create the dressing. Pour over the salad ingredients, and toss in the basil just before serving.

NUTRITION FACTS (per serving)	
Calories	124
Fat	6g
Carbohydrate	15g
Protein	4g

Note: Chiffonade is just a fancy way of saying chopped into long, thin strips. Stack the basil leaves, roll them up tightly, and slice them perpendicular to the roll.

Citrus Mint Quinoa Salad

YIELD: 4 SERVINGS

◐ GF

If you need a light, crisp recipe for a party, or just something to have in the refrigerator that's easy to add to any meal without taking the time to reheat, this Citrus Mint Quinoa Salad recipe is an easy, healthy go-to.

- 2 cups water
- 1 cup quinoa
- ¼ cup olive oil
- 2 lemons, juiced (about ¼ cup lemon juice)
- ½ cup scallions, chopped
- ½ cup peas (if frozen, thawed)
- 1 clove garlic, minced
- ¼ cup fresh mint, chopped
- ½ teaspoon sea salt

Directions
- In a medium saucepan, bring the water to a boil and add the quinoa. Reduce to simmer for about 18 to 20 minutes.
- When the quinoa is done, transfer it to a medium-size bowl. Add the olive oil and lemon juice and mix well.
- Add the remaining ingredients, except the mint and sea salt. Chill for at least 30 minutes before serving.
- Before serving, add the mint and sea salt. Mix well and serve.

NUTRITION FACTS (per serving)	
Calories	303
Fat	16g
Carbohydrate	32g
Protein	7g

Napa & Red Cabbage Salad

YIELD: 6 SERVINGS

If you want to take charge of your health, this cruciferous salad is a great place to start. Cabbage isn't just a great source of fiber, but also contains immune system boosting vitamins K, C and B_6. It's time to dig in.

- 1 head Napa cabbage, chopped into bite-size pieces
- ½ head red cabbage, chopped into bite-size pieces
- 1 ½ cups scallions, chopped
- 1 carrot, julienned
- ⅛ cup sesame seeds

Dressing
- ¼ cup water
- 2 tablespoons tahini, or unsweetened peanut butter
- 2 tablespoons olive oil
- 1 teaspoon honey
- 1 teaspoon gluten-free soy sauce

Directions
- In a large bowl, toss together the cabbages, scallions and carrots.
- In a small bowl, combine all the dressing ingredients and whisk thoroughly. Pour the dressing over the salad and toss gently. Sprinkle the sesame seeds on top before serving.

NUTRITION FACTS (per serving)	
Calories	150
Fat	9g
Carbohydrate	17g
Protein	4g

Quinoa Tabouli

YIELD: 6 SERVINGS

If you like traditional tabouli, then you'll love this version with a quinoa spin. Full of cleansing parsley, healthy fat and complex carbohydrates, this salad makes a great addition to any meal.

Salad
- 2 ½ cups parsley, chopped
- 6 scallions, diced
- ¼ cup fresh mint, chopped
- 1 cup diced tomato
- 2 cups cooked quinoa
- Sea salt, to taste

Dressing
- ¼ cup olive oil
- 2 lemons, juiced (about ¼ cup lemon juice)
- ½ teaspoon sea salt

Directions
- Combine the parsley, scallions, mint, tomato and quinoa in a large mixing bowl. Set aside.
- In a small bowl, combine all of the dressing ingredients and whisk thoroughly. Pour the dressing over the salad and toss to coat. Cover and let stand for at least one hour.
- Season with sea salt, if desired, upon serving.

NUTRITION FACTS (per serving)	
Calories	157
Fat	10g
Carbohydrate	12g
Protein	3g

Rainbow Kale Salad

YIELD: 8 SERVINGS

Every bite of this kale-packed salad will help you reduce bad (LDL) cholesterol, reduce inflammation and boost your immune system. The heartiness of the kale and cabbage makes this salad great for leftovers, too.

- 1 bunch kale, veins removed, coarsely chopped
- 3 cups red cabbage, shredded
- 1 yellow pepper, diced
- 1 small red onion, diced
- ¼ cup unsalted sunflower seeds, shelled
- ½ avocado, cubed

Dressing
- ¼ cup balsamic vinegar
- 2 lemons, juiced (¼ cup lemon juice)
- ¼ cup Dijon mustard
- ½ teaspoon sea salt

Directions
- Add all of the ingredients except the avocado and sunflower seeds to a large bowl.
- In a small bowl, combine all of the dressing ingredients and whisk thoroughly. Add the dressing to the salad and toss to coat.
- Just before serving, add the sunflower seeds and avocado.

NUTRITION FACTS (per serving)	
Calories	100
Fat	4g
Carbohydrate	12g
Protein	4g

Quinoa Lentil Salad

YIELD: 8 SERVINGS

Make this dish at the beginning of a busy week and keep in the refrigerator for a quick and healthy lunch.

- ½ cup green lentils
- ½ cup quinoa
- 2 tablespoons coconut oil
- 1 clove garlic, crushed
- ½ cup diced red pepper
- ¼ cup diced yellow onion
- ½ teaspoon sea salt

Directions

- In a medium saucepan, bring the green lentils to a boil in approximately 1 cup of water.
- In a separate pot, cook the quinoa in approximately 1 cup of water, adding coconut oil and garlic, for 18 to 20 minutes.
- Cook the lentils until they are soft, but not mushy, about 15 minutes. Remove them from the heat and strain out excess water in a colander.
- Add the peppers and onions to the quinoa and toss to properly combine. Finally, add in the cooked lentils. Toss one last time while sprinkling in sea salt. Serve warm or refrigerate for at least 30 minutes and up to 60 minutes before serving chilled.

NUTRITION FACTS (per serving)	
Calories	87
Fat	4g
Carbohydrate	10g
Protein	4g

Southwest Fajita Salad

YIELD: 4 SERVINGS

GF

Why wrap your fajitas in a tortilla shell when you can enjoy them over a big bed of lettuce loaded with your favorite toppings? Naturally anti-inflammatory bell peppers, onions, cumin and cayenne pepper give this recipe a kick.

- 1 ½ tablespoons coconut oil
- **For the Apple Eating Plan:** 1 pound skirt steak, lean, cut into thin 4- to 6-inch strips OR
- **For the Pear, Inverted Pyramid, Hourglass:** 1 pound grilled chicken, cut into thin 4- to 6-inch strips

- 1 orange bell pepper, sliced
- 1 red bell pepper, sliced
- 1 yellow bell pepper, sliced
- 1 medium yellow onion, sliced
- 1 clove garlic, diced
- 8 cups romaine lettuce, chopped

Seasoning

- 1 ½ teaspoons ground cumin
- ½ teaspoon cayenne pepper
- ½ teaspoon dried oregano

- ½ teaspoon potato starch (or corn starch)
- ½ teaspoon sea salt
- ½ cup water

Optional Sides

- 1 cup shredded cheddar or queso Chihuahua cheese
- 1 to 2 avocados, diced
- Chunky salsa

Directions

- Prepare the seasoning in advance by combining all of the ingredients in a small bowl. Whisk thoroughly and set aside.
- Heat a fajita pan or skillet over medium to high heat. Once the pan is hot, add the coconut oil and heat for at least 30 seconds. Add the meat and cook thoroughly.
- Add the peppers, onion and garlic and cook for 2 minutes until hot but still crunchy.
- Finally, add the seasoning and mix thoroughly. Remove the pan from the heat. Plate each serving over a bed of fresh lettuce, and sides if desired.

NUTRITION FACTS (per serving, not including sides)	
Calories	317
Fat	18g
Carbohydrate	7g
Protein	30g

Salads & Dressings

Cilantro Lime Vinaigrette

YIELD: 8 SERVINGS

This versatile dressing tastes great on any salad or as a marinade for chicken.

- 1 cup cilantro, lightly packed
- ½ cup olive oil
- ⅓ cup lime juice (from 2 limes)
- 2 tablespoons apple cider vinegar
- 2 tablespoons honey
- 1 clove garlic, crushed
- Pinch of sea salt

Directions
- Combine all of the ingredients in a blender and blend on high speed until smooth.
- Store and refrigerate in a sealed container for up to three months.

NUTRITION FACTS (per serving)	
Calories	142
Fat	12g
Carbohydrate	6g
Protein	0g

Almond & Honey-Crusted Pork Chops

YIELD: 4 SERVINGS

GF

Sweet and savory have come together beautifully in this protein-packed entrée. Pair this dish with Savory Sautéed Spinach (page 271) or a simple salad. These pork chops make for great leftovers, too! Dice up and add to a warm quinoa or vegetable-based dish.

- 4 thick-cut pork chops, about 4 ounces
- ½ cup almond meal
- ½ teaspoon sea salt
- ¼ cup honey

Directions
- Preheat oven to 375°F.
- Mix the sea salt and almond meal in a medium size bowl.
- Cover one side of the pork chops with a thin layer of honey.
- Dredge the honey-covered side in the almond meal mixture. Cover the opposite side of the pork chops with honey, and dredge in almond meal mixture.
- Place chops on ungreased baking sheet and bake for 25 to 30 minutes.

NUTRITION FACTS (per serving)	
Calories	221
Fat	5g
Carbohydrate	19g
Protein	25g

Entrées

Black Bean, Corn & Red Pepper Lettuce Wraps

YIELD: 4 SERVINGS

Leave the stove off and get ready to sink your teeth into these fiber-filled simple lettuce wraps that require no cooking whatsoever!

- 8 Bibb or Boston lettuce leaves
- 1 can black beans, drained and rinsed
- 1 cup corn, organic
- 1 red pepper, seeded and diced
- 2 limes, juiced
- 4 tablespoons olive oil
- Sea salt
- 1 avocado, sliced (optional)

Directions

- Wash and separate a few leaves of Bibb or Boston lettuce. Leave whole and set aside.
- Toss the beans, corn, peppers, lime juice and olive oil in a medium-size bowl. Season with sea salt as desired.
- Spoon the mixture into the lettuce leaves, adding avocado if desired. Fold like a taco and enjoy.

NUTRITION FACTS (per serving, not including avocado)	
Calories	277
Fat	13g
Carbohydrate	31g
Protein	9g

Black Bean & Quinoa Veggie Burgers

YIELD: 4 SERVINGS

For when you're craving a burger, but want a healthy break from the same old-same old.

- 1 can black beans, drained and rinsed
- 2 cups cooked quinoa
- ¼ cup oat flour
- 3 tablespoons olive oil, divided
- ¼ cup coarsely chopped red onion
- ¼ cup coarsely chopped cilantro

- 2 cloves garlic, minced
- ¾ teaspoon cumin
- ½ teaspoon sea salt
- ¼ teaspoon cayenne pepper
- ¼ teaspoon oregano
- 1 egg, lightly beaten

Directions

- Mash the black beans by hand in a medium-size bowl.
- Add the quinoa, oat flour and 1 tablespoon olive oil to black beans and mix well.
- Continue to mix in the red onions, cilantro, garlic, cumin, sea salt, cayenne pepper and oregano. Finally, add in the egg. Form four round patties, about 1 inch thick. Refrigerate for about one hour.
- Heat remaining olive oil in a skillet over low to medium heat.
- Add the patties to the skillet and cook for 5 to 7 minutes on each side, or until patties are golden brown.

NUTRITION FACTS (per serving)	
Calories	317
Fat	14g
Carbohydrate	37g
Protein	12g

Entrées

Cauliflower Crust Pizza

If you love pizza, but don't love all the doughy crust, then you've got to try this Cauliflower Crust Pizza. Load it up with your favorite ingredients and rest assured that you're getting a mouthful of flavor (and filling, nutritious veggies) in every bite.

- 6 cups water
- 1 head cauliflower, cut into large florets
- 2 eggs, lightly whisked
- ½ teaspoon dried sage, or 1 teaspoon fresh sage
- ½ teaspoon dried basil, or 1 teaspoon fresh basil
- ½ teaspoon dried oregano, or 1 teaspoon fresh oregano
- ½ teaspoon sea salt

Toppings
- Add your favorite pizza sauce (see note), and a few fresh toppings, like grilled chicken, fresh veggies, pineapple and a little mozzarella cheese.

Directions
- Preheat the oven to 400°F. Line a baking sheet with parchment paper. Set aside. Bring the water to a boil in a medium pot.
- Add the cauliflower florets to a food processor and process until the cauliflower is the consistency of rice. Scoop the cauliflower into the boiling water and cook for about 5 minutes.

- After the cauliflower is done, pour the pot's contents into a strainer. Using a large spoon, firmly press the cauliflower against the strainer to remove excess water.
- Spoon the cauliflower onto the center of a tea towel or cheesecloth to sit and cool momentarily. Pulling the ends of the towel over the cauliflower, squeeze the excess moisture out. Don't skip this step. If your cauliflower is too wet, you'll end up with a soggy crust.
- In a medium bowl, mix the cauliflower and eggs together. Finally, mix in the spices and sea salt. Expect the mixture to be somewhat runny.
- Scoop the mixture onto the parchment paper and form a circular crust about ½-inch thick. Bake for 35 to 40 minutes, or until the edges of the crust brown slightly.
- Add desired toppings and bake again for about 10 minutes.

NUTRITION FACTS (per serving, crust only)	
Calories	76
Fat	2g
Carbohydrate	8g
Protein	6g

Note: Looking to add a little variety to your pizza sauce? If you're going with a store-bought marinara or spaghetti sauce, make sure it doesn't contain high fructose corn syrup. If you want to make your own sauce, try spicing things up a bit by swapping the jarred sauce for the Sweet & Tangy BBQ Sauce recipe on page 279.

Lentil Burgers

YIELD: 6 SERVINGS

Lentils are a fantastic legume to cook with, especially when it comes to making veggie burgers. Filled with fiber and anti-inflammatory spices, this burger is simple, yet satisfying.

- 2 ½ cups water
- 1 teaspoon sea salt
- 1 tablespoon coconut oil, plus 1 teaspoon for greasing baking sheet
- ½ cup rice, rinsed and drained
- ½ cup red lentils, rinsed and drained
- 1 egg, whisked
- 1 carrot, shredded
- 1 clove garlic, crushed
- ¼ teaspoon ground turmeric
- ¼ teaspoon cumin

Directions

- Combine the water, salt, oil, rice and lentils in a large stockpot. Bring to a boil. Reduce heat and cook over low heat, uncovered, until water is absorbed, about 15 to 20 minutes. Remove from heat and allow to cool slightly.
- Preheat the oven to 400°F. Grease a baking sheet with coconut oil and set aside.
- In a medium mixing bowl, combine the egg, carrots, garlic, turmeric and cumin. After lentil mixture has cooled slightly, add to the egg mixture.
- Fold ingredients together. Divide the mixture evenly into six patties, about ½ inch thick. Place on the baking sheet and bake for approximately 24 minutes, flipping burgers halfway through.
- Serve with a salad topped with Belly Burn Cleanse Dressing (page 215), a side of avocado or steamed vegetables.

NUTRITION FACTS (per serving)	
Calories	157
Fat	4g
Carbohydrate	24g
Protein	6g

Lentil, Quinoa & Vegetable Stuffed Peppers

YIELD: 4 SERVINGS

Peppers make great serving bowls, especially when they're filled with the savory flavor of inflammation-fighting curry.

- 2 bell peppers (your choice of color)
- ¾ cup red lentils
- ½ cup quinoa
- 2 ⅓ tablespoons coconut oil, divided
- ½ teaspoon sea salt
- 2 ½ cups water
- ½ cup minced onion
- ½ cup thinly sliced carrots
- ½ cup chopped zucchini
- 1 clove garlic, crushed
- 1 teaspoon curry powder
- ¼ cup mozzarella cheese, shredded (optional)

Directions

- Cut the peppers in half lengthwise. Remove stems, membranes and seeds. Place on a baking sheet and set aside.
- Add the lentils, quinoa, 1 tablespoon of coconut oil, sea salt and the water to a stockpot and bring to a boil. Reduce heat and simmer until the water has been absorbed, approximately 15 minutes.
- At the same time, heat the remaining oil in a large pan. Add all of the vegetables and sauté. After the lentil/quinoa mixture is ready, add the curry powder. Next, add to the vegetable mixture and remove from heat. Mix thoroughly. Preheat the oven to 400°F.
- Spoon a generous amount of the mixture into each of the peppers. Sprinkle a little bit of cheese over the tops of each pepper, if desired. Bake for 15 to 20 minutes. Serve hot.

NUTRITION FACTS (per serving)	
Calories	294
Fat	10g
Carbohydrate	40g
Protein	13g

Entrées

Pot Pie Crumble

YIELD: 6 SERVINGS

An absolute home run in *The Belly Burn Plan*! The moment you taste this comfort food makeover, you'll never look at pot pie the same way again.

Filling
- 1 tablespoon coconut oil
- 1 ½ cups broccoli (fresh or frozen), chopped into florets
- ¾ cup thinly sliced carrots
- ½ cup minced onion
- ½ cup thinly sliced zucchini, green or yellow
- 1 tablespoon potato starch (or corn starch)
- ½ teaspoon sea salt
- 1 cup plus 2 tablespoons vegetable broth

Crumble Topping
- 1 ¼ cups almond flour
- 1 egg, lightly whisked
- 1 ½ tablespoons coconut oil

Directions

- To make the filling, heat the coconut oil in a medium skillet. Add the vegetables and sauté until cooked through.
- While the vegetables are cooking, whisk together the potato starch, sea salt and broth in a small bowl.
- Add the broth mixture to the cooked vegetables and bring to a boil. After mixture thickens, remove from heat. Pour mixture into a pie dish.
- Preheat the oven to 400°F.
- In a small bowl, combine the almond flour, egg and oil. The mixture will be thick and sticky. Mix it using a fork or your hands.
- Sprinkle the mixture over the top of the filling already in the pie dish. The topping will not cover the entire dish, rather appear as chunky crumbles on top.
- Bake for 15 to 20 minutes, or until crumble is golden brown.

NUTRITION FACTS (per serving)	
Calories	225
Fat	18g
Carbohydrate	14g
Protein	8g

Entrées

Shredded BBQ Chicken

YIELD: 6 SERVINGS

This meal is full of flavor, healthy spices and plenty of protein. Serve with Clean Cole Slaw (page 276) or a hearty leafy green salad. Looking for more kick in your BBQ sauce? Try my Sweet & Tangy BBQ Sauce (page 279).

- 1 ½ pounds chicken breasts
- ½ large onion, diced
- 6-ounce can tomato paste
- 28-ounce can diced tomatoes
- 3 cloves garlic, crushed
- 4 tablespoons apple cider vinegar
- 4 tablespoons honey
- 1 ½ tablespoons Worcestershire sauce
- 1-inch piece ginger, minced
- ½ teaspoon sea salt
- ½ teaspoon pepper
- ¼ teaspoon paprika
- ¼ teaspoon cayenne pepper

Directions

- Submerge the chicken breasts in a pot of water and bring to a boil. Cook until chicken is no longer pink through the middle, about 10-15 minutes. Remove from water and set aside.
- Begin making the BBQ sauce by combining the onions, tomato paste and diced tomatoes in a blender and blending until smooth before adding to a stockpot. Alternatively, if using an immersion blender, simply add the tomatoes and onions directly to the stockpot you'll be cooking with. Blend in the pot.
- Add all of the remaining ingredients to the stockpot and bring to a simmer.
- While the BBQ sauce is simmering, shred the chicken. Add the shredded chicken to the sauce and cook on the stovetop for 20 minutes. Serve warm.

NUTRITION FACTS (per serving)	
Calories	239
Fat	3g
Carbohydrate	24g
Protein	28g

Entrées

Chicken Vegetable Curry

YIELD: 6 SERVINGS

What else could be healthier and decrease inflammation more than a recipe that combines garlic, coconut milk, onion, curry and a rainbow of vegetables? Enjoy this Chicken Vegetable Curry for dinner and then again for lunch the next day. You'll never tire of this spice-filled classic.

- 1 tablespoon coconut oil
- 1 medium onion, diced
- 2 cloves garlic, crushed
- 1 pound chicken breasts (approximately 2-3), cubed
- 1 can unsweetened coconut milk
- 6 ounces tomato paste
- 1 cup water
- 2 teaspoons curry powder
- ½ teaspoon cayenne pepper
- ½ teaspoon sea salt
- 1 ½ teaspoons potato starch (or corn starch)
- 1 cup peas (frozen or fresh)
- 1 zucchini, thinly sliced
- 1 yellow squash, thinly sliced
- 8 ounces fresh mushrooms, sliced

Entrées

Directions

- In a stockpot, heat the coconut oil over medium heat. Add the onions and garlic, cooking until onions are translucent, about 4 or 5 minutes.
- Add the chicken and cook thoroughly, about 5 minutes. Add the coconut milk to the chicken. Bring to a simmer.
- In a separate bowl, combine the tomato paste and water until smooth. Add the curry powder, cayenne pepper, sea salt and potato starch. Whisk until dissolved. Add this mixture to the stockpot.
- After the tomato mixture is incorporated, add the remaining vegetables. Cook for an additional 12 to 15 minutes. Serve over brown rice, quinoa or enjoy on its own.

NUTRITION FACTS (per serving)	
Calories	272
Fat	14g
Carbohydrate	15g
Protein	23g

Chicken & Broccoli Stir-Fry

YIELD: 4 SERVINGS

GF

If you love getting Chinese take-out, but don't love all the processed oils and questionable seasonings, give this flavorful stir-fry a try. It's packed with plenty of fiber and protein, too.

- 2 tablespoons gluten-free soy sauce
- 2 tablespoons hoisin sauce
- ¼ cup rice wine vinegar
- 1 tablespoon potato starch (or corn starch)
- 2 cloves garlic, minced
- 2 teaspoons coconut oil, divided
- 4 cups broccoli florets
- 1 carrot, julienned
- ½ cup scallions
- 1 pound chicken breast, cut into 1-inch pieces

Directions
- In a small bowl, whisk together the soy sauce, hoisin sauce, rice wine vinegar, potato starch and garlic.
- Heat 1 teaspoon of the coconut oil in a large skillet. Add the broccoli, carrots and scallions, and sauté for about 2 minutes. Remove from the skillet and place in a large bowl.
- Add the remaining coconut oil to the skillet, then add the chicken and cook thoroughly.
- Re-add vegetable mixture to the skillet with the chicken, followed by the soy sauce mixture. Continue cooking until the soy mixture has thickened, about 2 minutes. Serve hot.

NUTRITION FACTS (per serving)	
Calories	180
Fat	5g
Carbohydrate	5g
Protein	26g

Curried Meatballs

YIELD: 6 SERVINGS (APPROXIMATELY 26 MEATBALLS)

With just a hint of curry, these meatballs will satisfy your taste buds without overwhelming them. Pair with a mixed greens salad and a side of warm rice for a quick and easy dinner tonight.

- 1 tablespoon olive oil, plus more for greasing baking sheet
- 1 pound lean ground turkey (organic preferred)
- 2 tablespoons yellow mustard
- ¼ teaspoon curry powder
- ¼ teaspoon ground turmeric
- ½ teaspoon sea salt
- ¼ cup old-fashioned oats

Directions
- Preheat the oven to 350°F. Grease a baking sheet with olive oil.
- In a medium-size bowl, combine the turkey, mustard and olive oil. Mix well.
- Next, add in the curry powder, turmeric and sea salt. When the color of the spices is evenly distributed, you'll know it's mixed enough. Lastly, add the oats and mix to combine.
- Divide the turkey mixture into small balls, about 1-inch round. Place them on the greased sheet and bake on the top rack for 13 minutes, turning halfway through, or until meatballs are lightly browned. (If your meatballs are larger than 1 inch, bake slightly longer.)

NUTRITION FACTS (per serving)	
Calories	136
Fat	9g
Carbohydrate	3g
Protein	14g

Quick Tip: You can make oat flour from old-fashioned oats. Simply grind them up in a clean coffee grinder and in about two minutes you'll end up with oat flour.

Spaghetti Squash with Turkey Bolognese

YIELD: 6 SERVINGS

GF

If you're looking for a great alternative to traditional spaghetti, you've found it. Spaghetti squash is a versatile and easy vegetable to cook, free of refined carbohydrates and has an easy, mild flavor that pleases all types of palates.

- 1 spaghetti squash
- 1 pound lean ground turkey (organic preferred)
- 2 cloves garlic, crushed
- 28-ounce can crushed tomatoes
- 6-ounce can tomato paste
- 1 tablespoon honey
- 3 tablespoons olive oil
- 2 teaspoons dried basil
- 2 teaspoons dried oregano
- ¼ teaspoon sea salt
- 1 tablespoon coconut oil

Directions

- Preheat the oven to 375°F. Fill a 9x13-inch pan with just under an inch of water. Set aside.
- Cut the spaghetti squash in half, lengthwise, and seed. Pierce the flesh with a fork a few times. Place the squash face down in pan and bake for 40 minutes.

- Brown the ground turkey in a skillet over medium heat, about 7 to 8 minutes, then add the garlic.
- While turkey is browning, combine crushed tomatoes, tomato paste, honey and olive oil in a medium-size bowl. Whisk thoroughly. Stir in the basil, oregano and sea salt. Add sauce to ground turkey and simmer for 10 to 15 minutes.
- You'll know the squash is done when you can easily stick a fork or knife through the flesh. When it's done, remove water from pan and carefully turn the squash over. It will be steaming hot, so use caution! Taking a fork or spoon, scrape the squash into a bowl. It should easily fall out—resembling spaghetti.
- Add the coconut oil to the squash and toss until the oil melts. Coconut oil solidifies in cold weather, but melts quickly at warm temps. Add sea salt to taste.
- By now your Bolognese sauce should be done. Serve the sauce over the squash and enjoy.

NUTRITION FACTS (per serving)	
Calories (per serving)	276
Fat	13g
Carbohydrate	23g
Protein	17g

Entrées

Sweet Potato Turkey Burgers

YIELD: 6 SERVINGS

If you like turkey burgers, you'll love these! The star of these
burgers is the sweet potato, which adds plenty of flavor
and texture.

- 2 tablespoons olive oil, divided
- 1 cup small cubed sweet potato
- 2 cloves garlic, crushed
- ¼ teaspoon sea salt
- ½ teaspoon curry powder
- 1 pound lean ground turkey (organic preferred)

Directions

- Preheat the oven to 350°F.
- In a medium skillet, heat 1 tablespoon of olive oil. Add the sweet
  potatoes and sauté for 5 to 7 minutes, or until soft in the middle.
  Remove from heat. Set aside.
- In a large mixing bowl, combine the garlic, sea salt, curry powder
  and remaining olive oil. Whisk quickly. Add the ground turkey
  and combine thoroughly. Fold in the sweet potato cubes.
- Form the mixture into six patties. Bake on a lightly greased
  cookie sheet for 12 to 17 minutes, turning once, or throw on the
  grill, cooking 6 to 7 minutes on each side.

NUTRITION FACTS (per serving)	
Calories	182
Fat	11g
Carbohydrate	7g
Protein	14g

Thai Turkey Lettuce Cups

YIELD: 4 SERVINGS (2 LETTUCE CUPS PER SERVING)

If you want to eat something with an Asian flair, but are bored with stir-fries, then it's time you tried these Thai Turkey Lettuce Cups. Served in edible cups made from lettuce, this entrée takes no time to make!

- 2 tablespoons olive oil or coconut oil
- 1 pound lean ground turkey (organic preferred)
- 1 cup shiitake mushrooms, stemmed and diced
- ¾ cup scallions, sliced
- 1 medium carrot, thinly sliced
- 1-inch piece ginger, diced
- 1 clove garlic, crushed
- ¼ cup hoisin sauce
- 2 tablespoons soy sauce (gluten-free)
- 8 Bibb or Boston lettuce leaves

Directions

- In a large skillet, heat the oil over medium heat. Add the ground turkey and brown, about 7 to 8 minutes.
- Add mushrooms, scallions, carrots, ginger, garlic, hoisin sauce and soy sauce. Continue to sauté over medium heat with the turkey until the carrots are slightly cooked, but still crunchy, about 5 minutes.
- Serve in lettuce cups and enjoy.

NUTRITION FACTS (per serving)	
Calories	304
Fat	15g
Carbohydrate	16g
Protein	21g

Taco Style Turkey Sloppy Joes

YIELD: 6 SERVINGS (2 LETTUCE CUPS PER SERVING)

GF

This high-protein recipe is easy on refined carbs and full of flavor. The classic comfort flavor of a traditional sloppy joe comes through served with the function of leafy greens. Forget the empty calories of the bun and enjoy with roasted vegetables or a side of rice instead.

- 1 tablespoon coconut oil
- ¼ cup chopped onion
- 1 pound lean ground turkey (organic preferred)
- ½ cup ketchup (organic)
- 3 tablespoons Sweet & Tangy BBQ Sauce (page 279)
- 1 tablespoon yellow mustard
- 1 tablespoon apple cider vinegar
- 1 ½ teaspoons Worcestershire sauce
- ½ teaspoon celery seed
- ¼ teaspoon pepper
- 12 Bibb or Boston lettuce leaves

Directions

- Heat a skillet over medium heat. Add the coconut oil once the skillet is warm. Add the onions to the heated oil and sauté for 3 to 4 minutes.
- Add the ground turkey to the skillet, stirring occasionally until thoroughly cooked, about 7 to 8 minutes.
- In a small bowl, mix together the remaining ingredients, except the lettuce, before adding to the turkey and onion mixture. Simmer for about 10 minutes.
- Serve "taco style" in lettuce leaves.

NUTRITION FACTS (per serving)	
Calories	161
Fat	8g
Carbohydrate	8g
Protein	14g

Turkey-Stuffed Peppers

YIELD: 6 SERVINGS

GF

Nothing could be more convenient when you're eating healthy than serving an entrée in an edible bowl made of a bell pepper! Dig in today and refrigerate leftovers for an easy-to-pack lunch tomorrow.

- 3 bell peppers (your choice of color)
- 1 tablespoon coconut oil
- 1 pound lean ground turkey (organic preferred)
- 2 cloves garlic, crushed
- 1 ½ cups marinara sauce (see Note)
- ¼ teaspoon sea salt
- ¼ teaspoon ground oregano
- 1 cup brown rice, cooked
- ½ cup mozzarella cheese, shredded
- **For the Hourglass Meal Plan:** Omit cheese

Directions

- Preheat oven to 375°F.
- Cut the bell peppers in half lengthwise. Remove stems, membranes and seeds. Place on an ungreased baking sheet and set aside.
- In a medium saucepan, heat the coconut oil, then add the ground turkey and brown thoroughly.
- Add the garlic, marinara sauce, sea salt and oregano to the cooked turkey. Simmer for 5 minutes.
- Add the rice to the turkey mixture. Mix thoroughly and remove from heat.
- Fill each pepper half with turkey mixture, then sprinkle cheese over the top.
- Bake for 20 minutes, or until cheese is golden brown.

NUTRITION FACTS (per serving)	
Calories	241
Fat	10g
Carbohydrate	14g
Protein	24g

Note: Be sure to choose a marinara sauce with no high-fructose corn syrup included.

Entrées

One-Pot Turkey Vegetable Chili

YIELD: 6 SERVINGS

GF

Get a full serving of vegetables and a healthy dose of protein in this quick and easy one-pot chili. Throw all the ingredients into one stockpot before a short workout and come back to a satisfying meal.

- 1 ½ tablespoons coconut oil
- 1 pound lean ground turkey (organic preferred)
- 2 (14.5-ounce) cans crushed tomatoes
- 2 carrots, chopped
- 1 medium yellow onion, chopped
- 1 ½ cups chopped mushrooms
- 1 zucchini, chopped
- 1 yellow pepper, chopped
- 2 stalks celery, chopped
- 2 cloves garlic, minced

Chili Seasoning
- 2 tablespoons paprika
- 1 teaspoon oregano
- 1 ½ teaspoons cumin
- 1 ½ teaspoons garlic powder
- ¾ teaspoon onion powder
- ¾ teaspoon cayenne pepper
- 1 teaspoon curry powder (optional)

Optional Toppings
- 1 avocado, cubed
- ½ cup sliced scallions
- ½ cup cilantro

Directions
- Heat the coconut oil in a stockpot. Add the ground turkey and cook until brown, stirring regularly, about 7 to 8 minutes.
- After the turkey has browned, add the tomatoes, vegetables, garlic and chili seasoning. Bring all of the ingredients to a simmer and cook over medium heat for 20 to 30 minutes.
- Serve warm, topped with your choice of avocado, scallions or cilantro.

NUTRITION FACTS (per serving, not including toppings)	
Calories	232
Fat	9g
Carbohydrate	22g
Protein	16g

Quick Tip: Get creative with paprika by sprinkling it on roasted vegetables or on omelets for a smoky flavor.

Soups & Sides

Cauliflower Soup

YIELD: 4 SERVINGS

This simple and healthy soup can be prepared in under 20 minutes. The Cauliflower Soup has a smooth texture and tastes great on its own, or with a hearty salad.

- 1 tablespoon coconut oil
- ½ cup chopped yellow onion
- 1 head cauliflower, cut into florets
- 4 cups vegetable broth
- 3 cloves garlic, crushed
- Sea salt, to taste

Directions
- In a medium stockpot, heat the coconut oil over medium heat.
- Add the onions, cooking until translucent (about 4 to 5 minutes).
- Add the cauliflower, broth and garlic. Bring to a boil, then reduce to a simmer. Cook, uncovered, until cauliflower can be pierced with a fork, approximately 7 to 8 minutes. Remove the pot from the heat.
- If using an immersion blender, blend directly in the pot until all ingredients are smooth. If using a blender, carefully add the hot ingredients and blend on high until all ingredients are smooth. Salt to taste before serving.

NUTRITION FACTS (per serving)	
Calories	104
Fat	3.5g
Carbohydrate	9g
Protein	3.5g

Chickpea & Lentil Soup

YIELD: 4 SERVINGS

Despite that I made this on a hot July day, I know it will be a standby in my kitchen this winter . . . or any time of year. Paired with the rich flavor of the browned onions, carrots and garlic, the lentils and chickpeas together make a great combination.

- 1 tablespoon coconut oil
- ½ cup chopped onions
- ½ cup sliced carrots
- 1 clove garlic, crushed
- 4 cups vegetable stock
- 1 can garbanzo beans (chickpeas), rinsed and drained
- ¾ cup red lentils
- Sea salt, to taste

Directions
- In a medium stockpot, heat the coconut oil over medium heat, then add the onions and carrots.
- After gently sautéing the vegetables for 3 to 4 minutes, add the garlic and sauté for 1 more minute.
- Add the stock, chickpeas and lentils to the mixture. Bring to a boil then reduce to a simmer.
- Cook over medium heat for 15 to 20 minutes, uncovered, or until lentils are cooked. Remove from heat, salt to taste and serve with a big leafy green salad.

NUTRITION FACTS (per serving)	
Calories	268
Fat	6g
Carbohydrate	41g
Protein	15g

Soups & Sides

Sautéed Lemon & Garlic Kale

YIELD: 4 SERVINGS

If you're not already making kale a staple in your grocery cart, this recipe is bound to change things. It's simple *and* delicious . . . not to mention incredibly healthy. With just a few ingredients, you'll be able to make this savory side dish in 10 minutes or less.

- 1 bunch kale, veins removed, coarsely chopped
- 2 tablespoons olive oil
- 2 cloves garlic, minced
- 2 tablespoons lemon juice
- Sea salt, to taste

Directions
- Heat the olive oil in a skillet over medium heat.
- Once the oil is hot, add the minced garlic. Sauté for about 30 seconds.
- Add the kale, continuously tossing until it begins to wilt, about 2 minutes.
- Add the lemon juice and continue to cook for another minute.
- Remove from heat, then sprinkle with a dash of sea salt and serve.

NUTRITION FACTS (per serving)	
Calories	96
Fat	7g
Carbohydrate	6g
Protein	2g

Savory Sautéed Spinach

YIELD: 4 SERVINGS

GF

This warm recipe will satisfy your craving for something on the salty side. Best of all, you don't need to spend a lot of preparation or cooking time in the kitchen to pull off this easy side dish!

- 1 tablespoon olive oil
- 3 strips uncured bacon, cut into ½-inch pieces widthwise
- 2 cloves garlic, minced
- 12 loosely packed cups baby spinach
- 2 tablespoons balsamic vinegar
- Sea salt, to taste

Directions

- In a large skillet, heat the olive oil over medium heat.
- Add the bacon and cook until crisp. Remove and set aside on a paper towel–lined plate.
- Add the garlic and cook for 1 minute.
- Slowly begin to add the spinach. As the spinach begins to wilt in the heat, add a little more until all of the spinach has been added to the skillet.
- Remove from heat and toss in the bacon, then the vinegar.
- Sprinkle with sea salt and serve.

NUTRITION FACTS (per serving)	
Calories	89
Fat	5g
Carbohydrate	6g
Protein	5g

Soups & Sides

Simple Butternut Squash Soup

YIELD: 4 SERVINGS

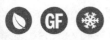

A great source of both potassium and vitamin B$_6$, butternut squash takes center stage in this simple, smooth recipe.

- 1 butternut squash, halved, seeded and peeled (see Note)
- 1 medium onion
- 4 cups vegetable broth or water
- 1 tablespoon coconut oil
- ½ teaspoon cumin
- ¼ teaspoon cayenne pepper
- Sea salt (optional)

Directions

- Coarsely chop the butternut squash and onion into 2-inch chunks.
- In a medium stockpot, combine all of the ingredients. Bring to a boil and heat until squash is soft, about 10 minutes. Remove from the heat. If using an immersion blender, blend directly in the pot until smooth. If using an upright blender, carefully add the hot ingredients, filling only halfway, and puree. Repeat with remaining liquid. If needed, add a pinch of sea salt before serving.

Note: Butternut squash come in varying sizes. Larger squash require additional broth to ensure the squash is completely submerged in liquid when cooking.

NUTRITION FACTS (per serving)	
Calories	191
Fat	4g
Carbohydrate	36g
Protein	3g

Split Pea & Turkey Soup

YIELD: 8 SERVINGS

Don't settle for canned soup loaded with preservatives when you can make your own nutritious version at home. If you're not cooking for eight, this soup freezes well and makes for great leftovers, too!

- 3 tablespoons coconut oil
- 1 onion, coarsely chopped
- 1 carrot, chopped
- 2 cups split peas
- 2 cups turkey breast, diced
- 1 sweet potato, cubed
- 3 cloves garlic, minced
- 2 teaspoons thyme (dried), or 1 tablespoon fresh thyme (minced)
- 1 teaspoon sea salt
- 8 cups vegetable broth

Directions
- Heat the coconut oil in a stockpot over medium heat. Add the onions and carrots. Sauté until the onions are translucent, about 4 to 5 minutes.
- Add the remaining ingredients. Bring to a boil for 10 minutes with the lid off. Reduce heat and simmer for 50 minutes with the lid on.
- If using an immersion blender, blend directly in the pot until the desired consistency is reached. If using an upright blender, carefully add the hot ingredients, filling only halfway, and blend on high until the desired consistency is reached. Repeat with remaining liquid, leaving a few chunks of vegetables for a nice texture. If needed, add a pinch of sea salt before serving.

NUTRITION FACTS (per serving)	
Calories	308
Fat	6g
Carbohydrate	38g
Protein	25g

Orange & Green Quinoa

YIELD: 4 SERVINGS

Get lots of color, crunch and flavor in this nutrient-dense quinoa dish. Asparagus is one of the greatest inflammation-fighting vegetables out there. Teamed up with the health benefits of carrots, this simple side works well as a warm accompaniment with dinner or chilled and sprinkled over a mixed greens salad for lunch.

- 1 tablespoon coconut oil
- 3 carrots, chopped in thin circles
- 6 asparagus spears, chopped in ½-inch pieces (throw out the ends)
- 2 cups vegetable broth or water
- 1 cup quinoa
- Sea salt (optional)

Directions

- In a large saucepan, melt coconut oil over medium heat. Add carrots and asparagus. Sauté for 3 to 5 minutes.
- Add the broth and quinoa to the pan and bring to a boil. Reduce heat to simmer. Cover for approximately 15 minutes, or until quinoa has absorbed all liquid.
- If preparing with water, add sea salt before serving, if desired.

Quick Tip: Quinoa comes in three different varieties: red, white and black. Most people are familiar with white. Red and black have similar nutritional properties, but they also take a little longer to cook. If you plan on using red or black quinoa, make sure to simmer on a low heat and allow for a little extra time.

NUTRITION FACTS (per serving)	
Calories	217
Fat	6g
Carbohydrate	31g
Protein	9g

Roasted Parsnips & Carrots

YIELD: 8 SERVINGS

Sometimes the simplest ingredients make the best dishes. Parsnips and carrots are no exception. Both are an excellent source of fiber, helping improve digestion and making you feel fuller longer.

- 1 ½ pounds parsnips, thinly sliced
- 1 pound carrots, thinly sliced
- ¼ cup olive oil
- ¼ cup parsley, chopped
- Sea salt, to taste

Directions
- Preheat the oven to 350°F.
- In a large mixing bowl, toss together the vegetables with the olive oil. Transfer to a roasting pan and bake for 45 minutes, or until vegetables are tender.
- Toss in the fresh parsley, sprinkle with sea salt and serve.

NUTRITION FACTS (per serving)	
Calories	127
Fat	7g
Carbohydrate	15g
Protein	1g

Soups & Sides

Clean Cole Slaw

Simple, delicious and clean are a few words that describe this cole slaw that pairs well with just about anything on the grill.

- 4 cups shredded cabbage (green)
- 3 medium or 2 large carrots, shredded
- ¼ cup olive oil
- ¼ cup apple cider vinegar
- 2 tablespoons honey
- ½ teaspoon mustard seed
- ½ teaspoon celery seed
- ¼ teaspoon sea salt

Directions
- Place the shredded cabbage and carrots in a bowl and set aside.
- In a small bowl, mix remaining ingredients.
- Pour the olive oil mixture over cabbage and carrots. Toss until thoroughly coated.
- Refrigerate for 20 to 30 minutes before serving.

NUTRITION FACTS (per serving)	
Calories	124
Fat	9g
Carbohydrate	10g
Protein	1g

Avocado Cilantro Dip

YIELD: 8 SERVINGS

This dip can be enjoyed with fresh vegetables or as a topping for a Tex-Mex-style salad.

- 2 avocados
- 1 clove garlic, crushed
- ⅓ cup plain yogurt
- ½ lime, juiced
- ½ teaspoon cayenne pepper
- ½ teaspoon cumin
- ¼ teaspoon sea salt
- ½ cup freshly chopped cilantro

Directions

- Combine all of the ingredients in a blender and blend on high speed until mixture is smooth and creamy.

NUTRITION FACTS (per 2 tablespoon serving)	
Calories	78
Fat	6g
Carbohydrate	6g
Protein	2g

Quick Tip: Looking for a better way to peel garlic that won't leave your fingers smelling, well . . . garlicky? Simply put a clove on a cutting board or flat surface. Place the flat side of a knife on the clove and press (or smash) firmly. The skin peels right off and your fingernails stay garlic-free.

Soups & Sides

Spicy Black Bean Dip

YIELD: 8 SERVINGS

Hummus isn't the only dip that works great with vegetables. Transform a regular old can of black beans into a healthy dip with a kick!

- 15-ounce can black beans, rinsed and drained
- 2 tablespoons tahini, or unsweetened peanut butter
- ¼ cup olive oil
- ¼ cup water
- 1 lime, juiced, or about 2 tablespoons
- 1 teaspoon cayenne pepper (see Note)
- ½ teaspoon cumin
- ¼ teaspoon sea salt

Directions
- Combine all of the ingredients in a blender and blend on high speed until texture is smooth. Refrigerate for at least 30 minutes before serving.

NUTRITION FACTS (per 2 tablespoon serving)	
Calories	138
Fat	8g
Carbohydrate	10g
Protein	6g

Note: Add cayenne pepper to suit the level of heat you desire.

Sweet & Tangy BBQ Sauce

YIELD: 6 SERVINGS

Even if you use this sauce only once in a while, it stores well for several months and makes a great addition to burgers, chicken or steak. I even use mine for dipping roasted vegetables.

- 1 cup ketchup (organic)
- ½ cup apple cider vinegar
- ½ cup honey
- 2 tablespoons Worcestershire sauce
- 1 tablespoon mustard seed powder
- ½ teaspoon sea salt

Directions

- Combine all of the ingredients in a medium bowl and whisk vigorously.
- Pour into a glass container, such as a mason jar, seal and shake. Store in your refrigerator until ready to use.

NUTRITION FACTS (per 2 tablespoon serving)	
Calories	88
Fat	0g
Carbohydrate	22g
Protein	0g

Quick Tip: Don't have a mason jar? Don't worry! Old applesauce, pickle or jam jars make a great substitute.

Chia Chocolate Pudding

YIELD: 8 SERVINGS

This recipe sounds really decadent, but it's full of healthy ingredients, including fiber, omega-3 fatty acids, antioxidants and much more. It stores well in a sealed container for up to 3 days.

- 2 cups unsweetened coconut milk
- ⅓ cup honey
- ½ cup cocoa, unsweetened
- ½ cup chia seeds

Directions
- Combine the coconut milk and honey in a medium bowl. Whisk until smooth.
- Slowly add the cocoa to the coconut milk mixture, whisking continuously until all the cocoa is dissolved.
- Finally, add the chia seeds, whisking until you have a smooth mixture.
- Refrigerate for at least two hours to set. If you're planning on serving this as a dessert to multiple people, pour into individual serving bowls before setting.

NUTRITION FACTS (per serving)	
Calories	135
Fat	6g
Carbohydrate	21g
Protein	4g

No Bake Chocolate Energy Balls

YIELD: 24 BALLS

The next time you need a sweet, guilt-free treat, turn to this recipe. Easy to make, these energy balls will get you in and out of the kitchen in less than 15 minutes.

- 1 ½ cups old-fashioned oats
- ½ cup unsweetened cocoa
- ½ teaspoon cinnamon
- 1 banana, mashed
- ¼ cup coconut oil, melted
- ¼ cup almond butter
- ¼ cup dried dates, chopped (7 or 8 dates)

Directions

- In a medium bowl, combine the oats, cocoa and cinnamon. Mix well.
- In a smaller bowl, combine the mashed banana, coconut oil and almond butter. Mix well.
- Add the wet ingredients to the dry ingredients. Make sure all ingredients are blended thoroughly. Finally, add the dates.
- With your hands, roll the date mixture into small balls and place on a baking sheet. Refrigerate for 30 minutes before removing from baking sheet and placing in a covered bowl. Keep refrigerated.

NUTRITION FACTS (per ball)	
Calories	67
Fat	4g
Carbohydrate	7g
Protein	2g

Chocolate Chunk Avocado Cookies

YIELD: 30 COOKIES

🌿 **GF**

Need a little indulgence, but don't want the guilt? Give your belly *and* body something to be happy about with this low-sugar cookie. Take a break from butter and use avocado instead.

- 1 cup oat flour
- ½ cup almond flour
- ½ teaspoon baking soda
- 1 avocado, mashed
- ¼ cup applesauce

- ⅓ cup honey
- 1 egg, lightly whisked
- 1 (3.5-ounce) dark chocolate bar (at least 70 percent cocoa), chopped

Directions
- Preheat the oven to 375°F. Line two baking sheets with parchment paper.
- In a medium bowl, combine the flours and baking soda.
- In a smaller bowl, mix together the avocado, applesauce, honey and egg.
- Add the avocado mixture to the flour mixture. After the batter is well blended, add in the pieces of chocolate. Drop small dollops of cookie dough on the prepared baking sheets. Bake for 6 to 8 minutes, or until cookies start to wrinkle at the top. Allow to cool, then enjoy.

NUTRITION FACTS (per cookie)	
Calories	69
Fat	3.5g
Carbohydrate	8g
Protein	1.5g

Chocolate Coconut Crunch Cookies

YIELD: 30 COOKIES

Not all cookies are unhealthy, and this recipe is no exception. The combination of cocoa and coconut offers a rich, satisfying flavor without any refined sugar.

- ½ cup coconut flour
- ½ cup almond flour
- ¼ cup coconut flakes
- ½ cup unsweetened cocoa powder
- ⅛ cup cacao nibs (optional)
- ¼ teaspoon baking soda
- 1 egg, lightly whisked
- 1 teaspoon vanilla extract
- ½ cup coconut oil, melted
- ⅓ cup honey

Directions
- Preheat the oven to 375°F. Line two baking sheets with parchment paper.
- In a medium bowl, combine the flours, coconut flakes, cocoa powder, cacao nibs (if using) and baking soda. Set aside.
- In a smaller bowl, combine the egg, vanilla, coconut oil and honey. After wet ingredients are thoroughly mixed, add to dry ingredients, mixing thoroughly.
- Roll small balls from the dough, about the size of a ping-pong ball and place on prepared sheet. Press gently with the backside of a spoon to flatten slightly, just enough to depress the center of the unbaked cookie. Bake for 6 to 8 minutes. Allow to cool, then enjoy.

NUTRITION FACTS (per cookie)	
Calories	73
Fat	6g
Carbohydrate	6g
Protein	1.5g

Recommendations

Below are a few recommendations for supplements, juices and teas from *The Belly Burn Plan*. Even though the supplements below are commonly used, be sure to check with a medical practitioner if you have any question about use as it applies to your own personal health.

Supplements

Probiotics

- **Nutrition Now® PB8** (capsule form) NutritionNow.com
- **inner-ēco™** (liquid form) inner-eco.com
- **Garden of Life Primal Defense ULTRA** (capsule form) GardenOfLife.com

Omega-3 Fatty Acids

- **Nordic Naturals Arctic-D Cod Liver Oil®** (liquid form) NordicNaturals.com
- **Carlson® Norwegian Cod Liver Oil** (soft gels) CarlsonLabs.com
- **NOW® Foods Certified Organic Flax Seed Oil** (liquid form) NOWFoods.com

Protein Powders

- **tera'swhey® Protein Powder** (any flavor, whey-based) teraswhey.com
- **Vega™ Protein & Greens** (any flavor, vegetarian) MyVega.com

Juices and Teas

Pomegranate Juices

- **Lakewood® Organic Pure Pomegranate Juice** LakewoodJuices.com
- **Jarrow PomeGreat Pomegranate Juice** Jarrow.com

Herbal Teas

- **Traditional Medicinals®** (any herbal variety) TraditionalMedicinals.com
- **Yogi®** (any herbal variety) YogiProducts.com
- **Alvita®** (any herbal variety) Alvita.com

Endnotes

Chapter 1

1. Centers for Disease Control and Prevention. *National Diabetes Statistics Report*, 2014. National Diabetes Education Program. http://www.cdc.gov/diabetes/pubs/statsreport14/national-diabetes-report-web.pdf (accessed August 8, 2014).
2. Yang, Ronghua, and Lili A. Barouch. "Leptin Signaling and Obesity." *Circulation Research*. http://circres.ahajournals.org/content/101/6/545.abstract (accessed September 4, 2014).
3. Shapiro, Alexandra, Wei Mu, Carlos Roncal, Kit-Yan Cheng, Richard J. Johnson, and Philip J. Scarpace. "Fructose-induced Leptin Resistance Exacerbates Weight Gain in Response to Subsequent High-Fat Feeding." National Center for Biotechnology Information. http://www.ncbi.nlm.nih.gov/pmc/articles/PMC2584858/ (accessed August 4, 2014).
4. Bjørbæk, Christian. "Central Leptin Receptor Action and Resistance in Obesity." *Journal of Investigative Medicine* 7, no. 57 (2009): 789-794.
5. Lee, John R. *What Your Doctor May Not Tell You About Premenopause*. New York: Grand Central Publishing, 1999.
6. L. Aksglaede. "The Sensitivity of the Child to Sex Steroids: Possible Impact of Exogenous Estrogens." *Human Reproduction Update* 12, no. 4 (2006): 341-349.
7. Axon, Andrew, Felicity E. b. May, Luke E. Gaughan, Faith M. Williams, Peter G. Blain, and Matthew C. Wright. "Tartrazine and Sunset Yellow are Xenoestrogens in a New Screening Assay to Identify Modulators of Human Oestrogen Receptor Transcriptional Activity." *Toxicology* 298, no. 1-3 (2012): 40-51.
8. Lucero, Jennifer, Bernard L. Harlow, Robert L. Barbieri, Patrick Sluss, and Daniel W. Cramer. "Early Follicular Phase Hormone

Levels in Relation to Patterns of Alcohol, Tobacco, and Coffee Use." *Fertility and Sterility* 76, no. 4 (2001): 723-729.

9. Phrakonkham, Pascal, Say Viengchareun, Christine Belloir, Marc Lombès, Yves Artur, and Marie-Chantal Canivenc-Lavier. "Dietary Xenoestrogens Differentially Impair 3T3-L1 Preadipocyte Differentiation and Persistently Affect Leptin Synthesis." *The Journal of Steroid Biochemistry and Molecular Biology* 110, no. 1-2 (2008): 95-103.

10. B. A. Lessey and Young S. L. "Homeostasis Imbalance in the Endometrium of Women with Implantation Defects: The Role of Estrogen and Progesterone." *Seminars in Reproductive Medicine* 32, no. 5 (2014): 365-375.

11. Upson, K., S. Sathyanarayana, AJ De Roos, HM Koch, D. Scholes, and VL Holt. "A Population-based Case-control Study of Urinary Bisphenol A Concentrations and Risk of Endometriosis." *Human Reproduction* 29, no. 11 (2014): 2457-64.

12. Darbre, P. D., A. Aljarrah, W. R. Miller, N. G. Coldham, M. J. Sauer, and G. S. Pope. "Concentrations Of Parabens In Human Breast Tumours." *Journal of Applied Toxicology* 24, no. 1 (2004): 5-13.

13. Arrebola, Juan P., José Pumarega, Magda Gasull, Mariana F. Fernandez, Piedad Martin-Olmedo, José M. Molina-Molina, María Fernández-Rodríguez, Miquel Porta, and Nicolás Olea. "Adipose Tissue Concentrations of Persistent Organic Pollutants and Prevalence of Type 2 Diabetes in Adults from Southern Spain." *Environmental Research* 122 (2013): 31-37.

14. King, Frank J. "Anti-Aging, Homeopathy, and HGH." *The American Chiropractor.* http://www.theamericanchiropractor.com/ articles-special-feature/5787-anti-aging-homeopathy-and-hgh.html (accessed August 4, 2014).

Chapter 2

1. Irving, Brian A., Christopher K. Davis, David W. Brock, Judy Y. Weltman, Damon Swift, Eugene J. Barrett, Glenn A. Gaesser, and Arthur Weltman. "Effect of Exercise Training Intensity on Abdominal Visceral Fat and Body Composition." *Medicine & Science in Sports & Exercise* 40, no. 11 (2008): 1863-1872.

2. Centers for Disease Control and Prevention. "Americans Slightly Taller, Much Heavier Than Four Decades Ago." http://www.cdc.gov/nchs/pressroom/04news/americans.htm (accessed September 10, 2014).

3. Davis, W. J, D. T. Wood, R. G. Andrews, L. M. Elkind, and W. B. Davis. "Concurrent Training Enhances Athletes' Strength, Muscle Endurance, and Other Measures." *Journal of Strength and Conditioning Research* 5 (2008): 1487-1502.

4. American Academy of Orthopaedic Surgeons. "Lifetime of Fitness: Fountain of Youth for Bone, Joint Health?" *ScienceDaily.* www.sciencedaily.com/releases/2014/08/140827122634.htm (accessed August 28, 2014).

5. Heijden, Gert-Jan Van Der, Zhiyue J. Wang, Zili Chu, Gianna Toffolo, Erica Manesso, Pieter J. J. Sauer, and Agneta L. Sunehag. "Strength Exercise Improves Muscle Mass and Hepatic Insulin Sensitivity in Obese Youth." *Medicine & Science in Sports & Exercise* 42, no. 11 (2010): 1973-1980.

6. Heydari, M., J. Freund, and S. H. Boutcher. "The Effect of High-Intensity Intermittent Exercise on Body Composition of Overweight Young Males." *Journal of Obesity* 2012 (2012): 1-8.

7. Skelly, L. E, P. C. Andrews, J. B. Gillen, B. J. Martin, M. E. Percival, and M. J. Gibala. "High-intensity Interval Exercise Induces 24-h Energy Expenditure Similar to Traditional Endurance Exercise Despite Reduced Time Commitment." *Applied Physiology, Nutrition & Metabolism* 39, no. 7 (2014): 845-8.

8. Stokes, Keith. "Growth Hormone Responses to Sub-Maximal and Sprint Exercise." Growth Hormone & IGF Research 13, no. 5 (2003): 225-238.

9. Little, J. P., J. B. Gillen, M. F. Percival, A. Safdar, M. A. Tarnopolsky, Z. Punthakee, M. E. Jung, and M. J. Gibala. "Low-volume High-Intensity Interval Training Reduces Hyperglycemia and Increases Muscle Mitochondrial Capacity in Patients with Type 2 Diabetes." *Journal of Applied Physiology* 111, no. 6 (2011): 1554-1560.

10. Gillen, J. B., J. P. Little, Z. Punthakee, M. A. Tarnopolsky, M. C. Riddell, and M. J. Gibala. "Acute High-Intensity Interval Exercise Reduces the Postprandial Glucose Response and Prevalence of

Hyperglycaemia in Patients with Type 2 Diabetes." *Diabetes, Obesity and Metabolism* 5 (2012): 575-7.

Chapter 3

1. "Kellogg's Nutri-Grain Fruit Crunch™ Granola Bars Strawberry Parfait." http://www.nutrigrain.com/product-detail.aspx?product=31274 (accessed September 1, 2014).
2. "PC Ice Cream Shop Flavours Mint Chocolate Ice Cream." http://www.presidentschoice.ca/en_CA/products/productlisting/pc_mint_chocolate_ice_creamprod850053.html (accessed September 8, 2014).
3. Profiling food consumption in America. In: US Department of Agriculture. *Agriculture Fact Book* 2001-2002. Washington, DC: US Government Printing Office; 13-21.
4. USDA Economic Research Service. "Wheat's Role in the U.S. Diet." http://www.ers.usda.gov/topics/crops/wheat/wheats-role-in-the-us-diet.aspx#. (accessed August 8, 2014).
5. "Sugar 101." Sugar 101. http://www.heart.org/HEARTORG/GettingHealthy/NutritionCenter/HealthyEating/Sugar-101_UCM_306024_Article.jsp (accessed August 8, 2014).
6. Avena, Nicole M., Pedro Rada, and Bartley G. Hoebel. "Evidence for Sugar Addiction: Behavioral and Neurochemical Effects of Intermittent, Excessive Sugar Intake." *Neuroscience & Biobehavioral Reviews* 32, no. 1 (2008): 20-39.
7. Howard, PhD, Barbara, and Judith Wylie-Rosett, RD, EdD. "Sugar and Cardiovascular Disease." *Sugar and Cardiovascular Disease.* http://circ.ahajournals.org/content/106/4/523.full (accessed August 9, 2014).
8. Nordestgaard, B. G., M. Benn, P. Schnohr, and A. Tybjaerg-Hansen. "Nonfasting Triglycerides and Risk of Myocardial Infarction, Ischemic Heart Disease, and Death in Men and Women." *JAMA: The Journal of the American Medical Association* 298, no. 3 (2007): 299-308.
9. Stanhope, Kimber L, and Peter J. Havel. "Fructose Consumption: Potential Mechanisms for Its Effects to Increase Visceral Adi-

posity and Induce Dyslipidemia and Insulin Resistance." *Current Opinion in Lipidology* 19, no. 1 (2008): 16-24.

10. Marchese, Michelle E, Rajesh Kumar, Laura A. Colangelo, Pedro C. Avila, David R. Jacobs, Myron Gross, Akshay Sood, Kiang Liu, and Joan M. Cook-Mills. "The Vitamin E Isoforms α-tocopherol and γ-tocopherol Have Opposite Associations with Spirometric Parameters: The CARDIA Study." *Respiratory Research* 15, no. 1 (2014): 31.

11. Henderson, Samuel T, Janet L. Vogel, Linda J. Barr, Fiona Garvin, Julie J. Jones, and Lauren C. Costantini. "Study of the Ketogenic Agent AC-1202 in Mild to Moderate Alzheimer's Disease: A Randomized, Double-Blind, Placebo-Controlled, Multicenter Trial." *Nutrition & Metabolism* 6, no. 1 (2009): 31.

12. Siri-Tarino, P. W, Q. Sun, F. B. Hu, and R. M. Krauss. "Meta-Analysis of Prospective Cohort Studies Evaluating the Association of Saturated Fat with Cardiovascular Disease." *American Journal of Clinical Nutrition* 91, no. 3 (2010): 535-546.

13. Wolk, A. "A Prospective Study of Association of Monounsaturated Fat and Other Types of Fat with Risk of Breast Cancer." *Archives of Internal Medicine* 158, no. 1 (1998): 41-45.

Chapter 4

1. Neumarksztainer, D, M. Wall, J. Guo, M. Story, J. Haines and M. Eisenberg. "Obesity, Disordered Eating, and Eating Disorders in a Longitudinal Study of Adolescents: How Do Dieters Fare 5 Years Later?" *Journal of the American Dietetic Association* 106, no. 4 (2006): 559-568.

2. Tomiyama, A. J., T. Mann, D. Vinas, J. M. Hunger, J. DeJager, and S. E. Taylor. "Low Calorie Dieting Increases Cortisol." *Psychosomatic Medicine* 72, no. 4 (2010): 357-364.

3. Fontana, L., J. C. Eagon, M. E. Trujillo, P. E. Scherer, and S. Klein. "Visceral Fat Adipokine Secretion Is Associated with Systemic Inflammation in Obese Humans." *Diabetes* 56, no. 4 (2007): 1010-1013.

4. Cifuentes, Mariana, Cecilia Albala, and Cecilia V Rojas. "Differences in Lipogenesis and Lipolysis in Obese and Non-Obese

Adult Human Adipocytes." *Biological Research* 41, no. 2 (2008): 1.

5. Zechner, Rudolf, Robert Zimmermann, Thomas O. Eichmann, Sepp D. Kohlwein, Guenter Haemmerle, Achim Lass, and Frank Madeo. "FAT SIGNALS—Lipases and Lipolysis in Lipid Metabolism and Signaling." *Cell Metabolism* 15, no. 3 (2012): 279-291.

6. McTernan, P. G., A. L. Harte, L. A. Anderson, A. Green, S. A. Smith, et al. "Insulin and Rosiglitazone Regulation of Lipolysis and Lipogenesis in Human Adipose Tissue In Vitro." *Diabetes* 51, no. 5 (2002): 1493-1498.

7. Jensen, M. D. "Role of Body Fat Distribution and the Metabolic Complications of Obesity." *Journal of Clinical Endocrinology & Metabolism* 93, no. 11_Supplement_1 (2008): s57-s63.

8. Rippe, James M. "Adipose Tissue." *Encyclopedia of Lifestyle Medicine & Health.* Thousand Oaks, Calif.: Sage Publications, 2012. 15.

9. Matsuzawa, Yuji, Iichiro Shimomura, Tadashi Nakamura, Yoshiaki Keno, Kasuaki Kotani, and Katsuto Tokunaga. "Pathophysiology and Pathogenesis of Visceral Fat Obesity." *Obesity Research* 3, no. S2 (1995): 187s-194s.

10. Centers for Disease Control and Prevention. "Obesity and Overweight." http://www.cdc.gov/nchs/fastats/obesity-overweight.htm (accessed September 23, 2014).

Chapter 5

1. Liau, Kai Ming, Yeong Yeh Lee, Chee Keong Chen, and Aida Hanum G. Rasool. "An Open-Label Pilot Study to Assess the Efficacy and Safety of Virgin Coconut Oil in Reducing Visceral Adiposity." *ISRN Pharmacology* 2011 (2011): 1-7.

2. Assunção, Monica L., Haroldo S. Ferreira, Aldenir F. dos Santos, Cyro R. Cabral, and Telma M. M. T. Florêncio. "Effects of Dietary Coconut Oil on the Biochemical and Anthropometric Profiles of Women Presenting Abdominal Obesity." *Lipids* 44, no. 7 (2009): 593-601.

3. Gavrieli, A., M. Yannakoulia, E. Fragopoulou, D. Margaritopoulos, J. P. Chamberland, P. Kaisari, S. A. Kavouras, and C. S. Mantzoros. "Caffeinated Coffee Does Not Acutely Affect Energy Intake, Appetite, or Inflammation but Prevents Serum Cortisol Concentrations

from Falling in Healthy Men." *Journal of Nutrition* 141, no. 4 (2011): 703-707.

4. Bennett, Jeanette M., Isabella M. Rodrigues, and Laura Cousino Klein. "Effects of Caffeine and Stress on Biomarkers of Cardiovascular Disease in Healthy Men and Women with a Family History of Hypertension." *Stress and Health* 29, no. 5 (2013): 401-409.

5. Siler, R. A. Neese and M. K. Hellerstein. "De Novo Lipogenesis, Lipid Kinetics, and Whole-Body Lipid Balances in Humans After Acute Alcohol Consumption." *American Journal of Clinical Nutrition* 70, no. 5 (1999): 928-936.

6. Venables, C. J. Hulston, H. R. Cox, and A. E. Jeukendrup. "Green Tea Extract Ingestion, Fat Oxidation, and Glucose Tolerance in Healthy Humans." *American Journal of Clinical Nutrition* 87, no. 3 (2008): 778-784.

7. Berlin, A. Grimaldi, C. Landault, F. Cesselin, and A. J. Puech. "Suspected Postprandial Hypoglycemia Is Associated with Beta-Adrenergic Hypersensitivity and Emotional Distress." *The Journal of Clinical Endocrinology & Metabolism* 79, no. 5 (1994): 1428-1433.

8. Mehran, Arya E., Susanne M. Clee, G. Stefano Brigidi, Nicole M. Templeman, James D. Johnson, Shernaz X. Bamji, Timothy J. Kieffer, Bradford G. Hoffman, Ali Asadi, Jose Diego Botezelli, Xiaoke Hu, Kwan-Yi Chu, and Gareth E. Lim. "Hyperinsulinemia Drives Diet-Induced Obesity Independently of Brain Insulin Production." *Cell Metabolism* 16, no. 6 (2012): 723-737.

Chapter 7

1. Ricci, Walter F. Stewart, Elsbeth Chee, Carol Leotta, Kathleen Foley, and Marc C. Hochberg. "Back Pain Exacerbations and Lost Productive Time Costs in United States Workers." *Spine* 31, no. 26 (2006): 3052-3060.

Chapter 8

1. Lovallo, William R., Noha H. Farag, Andrea S. Vincent, Terrie L. Thomas, and Michael F. Wilson. "Cortisol Responses to Mental Stress, Exercise, and Meals Following Caffeine Intake in Men

and Women." *Pharmacology Biochemistry and Behavior* 83, no. 3 (2006): 441-447.

2. Keijzers, G. B., B. E. De Galan, C. J. Tack, and P. Smits. "Caffeine Can Decrease Insulin Sensitivity in Humans ." Diabetes Care 25, no. 2 (2002): 364-369.

3. Nettleton, J. A., P. L. Lutsey, Y. Wang, J. A. Lima, E. D. Michos, and D. R. Jacobs. "Diet Soda Intake and Risk of Incident Metabolic Syndrome and Type 2 Diabetes in the Multi-Ethnic Study of Atherosclerosis (MESA)." *Diabetes Care* 32, no. 4 (2009): 688-694.

4. Rong, Y., L. Chen, T. Zhu, Y. Song, M. Yu, Z. Shan, A. Sands, F. B. Hu, and L. Liu. "Egg Consumption and Risk of Coronary Heart Disease and Stroke: Dose-Response Meta-Analysis of Prospective Cohort Studies." *BMJ* 346, no. jan07 2 (2013): e8539-e8539.

5. Thongprakaisang, Siriporn, Apinya Thiantanawat, Nuchanart Rangkadilok, Tawit Suriyo, and Jutamaad Satayavivad. "Glyphosate Induces Human Breast Cancer Cells Growth via Estrogen Receptors." *Food and Chemical Toxicology* 59 (2013): 129-136.

6. Koller, Verena J., Maria Fürhacker, Armen Nersesyan, Miroslav Mišík, Maria Eisenbauer, and Siegfried Knasmueller. "Cytotoxic and DNA-Damaging Properties of Glyphosate and Roundup in Human-Derived Buccal Epithelial Cells." *Archives of Toxicology* 86, no. 5 (2012): 805-813.

7. Imhof, Armin, Margit Froehlich, Hermann Brenner, Heiner Boeing, Mark B Pepys, and Wolfgang Koenig. "Effect of Alcohol Consumption on Systemic Markers of Inflammation." *The Lancet* 357, no. 9258 (2001): 763-767.

8. Yang, PhD, Zfeng Zhang, MD, PhD, Edward Gregg, PhD, W. Dana Flanders, MD, ScD, Robert Merritt, MA, and Frank Hu, MD, Phd. "Added Sugar Intake and Cardiovascular Diseases Mortality among US Adults." *JAMA Internal Medicine* 174, no. 4 (2014): 516-524.

9. Manzel, Arndt, Dominik N. Muller, David A. Hafler, Susan E. Erdman, Ralf A. Linker, and Markus Kleinewietfeld. "Role of 'Western Diet' in Inflammatory Autoimmune Diseases." *Current Allergy and Asthma Reports* 14, no. 1 (2014): 404.

10. Koning, L. De, V. S. Malik, M. D. Kellogg, E. B. Rimm, W. C. Willett, and F. B. Hu. "Sweetened Beverage Consumption, Incident Coro-

nary Heart Disease, and Biomarkers of Risk in Men." *Circulation* 125, no. 14 (2012): 1735-1741.

11. Master, Rachel, Angela Liese, Steven Haffner, Lynne Wagenknecht and Anthony Hanley. "Whole and Refined Grain Intakes Are Related to Inflammatory Protein Concentrations in Human Plasma." *The Journal of Nutrition* 140, no. 3 (2010): 587-594.

12. Simopoulos, A.P. "The Importance of the Ratio of Omega-6/Omega-3 Essential Fatty Acids." *Biomedicine & Pharmacotherapy* 56, no. 8 (2002): 365-379.

13. Marchese, Michelle E, Rajesh Kumar, Laura A. Colangelo, Pedro C. Avila, David R. Jacobs, Myron Gross, Akshay Sood, Kiang Liu, and Joan M. Cook-Mills. "The Vitamin E Isoforms α-tocopherol and γ-tocopherol Have Opposite Associations with Spirometric Parameters: The CARDIA Study." *Respiratory Research* 15, no. 1 (2014): 31.

Chapter 9

1. "In U.S., 40% Get Less Than Recommended Amount of Sleep." http://www.gallup.com/poll/166553/less-recommended-amount-sleep.aspx (accessed June 13, 2014).

2. Van Cauter, PhD, Eve, Kristen Knutson, PhD, Rachel Leproult, PhD, and Karine Spiegel, PhD. "The Impact of Sleep Deprivation on Hormones and Metabolism." http://www.medscape.org/viewarticle/502825 (accessed June 15, 2014).

3. Nedeltcheva, MD, MD, Arlet V., Jennifer M. Kilkus, MS, Jacqueline Imperial, RN, Dale A. Schoeller, and Plamen D. Penev, MD, PhD. "Insufficient Sleep Undermines Dietary Efforts to Reduce Adiposity." *Annals of Internal Medicine.* http://annals.org/article.aspx?articleid=746184 (accessed June 13, 2014).

4. Donga, Esther, Marieke Van Dijk, J. Gert Van Dijk, Nienke R. Biermasz, Gert-Jan Lammers, Klaas W. Van Kralingen, Eleonara P. M. Corssmit, and Johannes A. Romijn. "A Single Night of Partial Sleep Deprivation Induces Insulin Resistance in Multiple Metabolic Pathways in Healthy Subjects." *Endocrinology* 151, no. 5 (2010): 2399-2399.

5. University of Chicago Medical Center. "Even Your Fat Cells Need Sleep, According to New Research." www.sciencedaily.com/releases/2012/10/121015170822.htm (accessed June 13, 2014).
6. Spiegel, Karine. "Brief Communication: Sleep Curtailment in Healthy Young Men Is Associated with Decreased Leptin Levels, Elevated Ghrelin Levels, and Increased Hunger and Appetite." *Annals of Internal Medicine* 141, no. 11 (2004): 846.
7. Leproult, R., G. Copinschi, O. Buxton, and E. Van Cauter. "Sleep Loss Results in an Elevation of Cortisol the Next Evening." *Sleep* 10 (1997): 865-870
8. "Facts about Insomnia." http://sleepfoundation.org/insomnia/what-is-insomnia/facts/ (accessed July 2, 2014).
9. Drake, C, T. Roehrs, J. Shambroom, and T. Roth. "Caffeine Effects on Sleep Taken 0, 3, or 6 Hours before Going to Bed." *Journal of Clinical Sleep Medicine* 9, no. 11 (2013): 1195-1200.
10. Wood, Brittany, Mark S. Rea, Barbara Plitnick, and Mariana G. Figueiro. "Light Level and Duration of Exposure Determine the Impact of Self-Luminous Tablets on Melatonin Suppression." *Applied Ergonomics* 44, no. 2 (2013): 237-240.
11. National Sleep Foundation. "The Sleep Environment." http://sleepfoundation.org/sleep-news/the-sleep-environment (accessed July 5, 2014).
12. Ebrahim, Irshaad O., Colin M. Shapiro, Adrian J. Williams, and Peter B. Fenwick. "Alcohol and Sleep I: Effects on Normal Sleep." *Alcoholism: Clinical and Experimental Research* 37, no. 4 (2013): 539-549.
13. Naismith, SC, B. Hickie, Z. Tereping, S. M. Rajaratnam, J. R. Hodges, S. Bolitho, N. L. Rogers, and S. L. Lewis. "Circadian Misalignment and Sleep Disruption in Mild Cognitive Impairment." *Journal of Alzheimer's Disease* 38, no. 4 (2014): 857-866.
14. Falchi, Fabio, Pierantonio Cinzano, Christopher D. Elvidge, David M. Keith, and Abraham Haim. "Limiting the Impact of Light Pollution on Human Health, Environment and Stellar Visibility." *Journal of Environmental Management* 92, no. 10 (2011): 2714-2722.

Chapter 10

1. Sominsky, Luba, and Sarah J. Spencer. "Eating Behavior and Stress: A Pathway to Obesity." *Frontiers in Psychology* 5 (2014): 434.

2. Epel, Elissa, Rachel Lapidus, Bruce Mcewen, and Kelly Brownell. "Stress May Add Bite to Appetite in Women: A Laboratory Study of Stress-Induced Cortisol and Eating Behavior." *Psychoneuroendocrinology* 26, no. 1 (2001): 37-49.

3. Rada, P., N. M. Avena, and B. G. Hoebel. "Daily Bingeing on Sugar Repeatedly Releases Dopamine in the Accumbens Shell." *Neuroscience* 134, no. 3 (2005): 737-744.

4. Colantuoni, Carlo, Pedro Rada, Joseph McCarthy, Caroline Patten, Nicole M. Avena, Andrew Chadeayne and Bartley G. Hoebel. "Evidence That Intermittent, Excessive Sugar Intake Causes Endogenous Opioid Dependence." *Obesity* 10, no. 6 (2002): 478-488.

5. Epel, ES, N. McEwen, T. Seeman, K. Matthews, G. Castellazzo, K. D. Brownell, J. Bell, and J. R. Ickovics. "Stress and Body Shape: Stress-Induced Cortisol Secretion Is Consistently Greater Among Women with Central Fat." *Psychosomatic Medicine* 62, no. 5 (2000): 623-632.

6. "Stress and Eating." http://www.apa.org. http://www.apa.org/news/press/releases/stress/2013/eating.aspx (accessed June 5, 2014).

7. Lovallo, William R., Noha H. Farag, Andrea S. Vincent, Terrie L. Thomas, and Michael F. Wilson. "Cortisol Responses to Mental Stress, Exercise, and Meals Following Caffeine Intake in Men and Women." *Pharmacology Biochemistry and Behavior* 83, no. 3 (2006): 441-447.

8. Gragnoli, C. "Hypothesis of the Neuroendocrine Cortisol Pathway Gene Role in the Comorbidity of Depression, Type 2 Diabetes, and Metabolic Syndrome." *The Application of Clinical Genetics* 7 (2014): 43-53.

9. Björntorp. P. "Do Stress Reactions Cause Abdominal Obesity and Comorbidities?" *Obesity Review* 2 (2001): 73-86.

10. Nicolaides, Nicolas C., Elli Kyratzi, Agaristi Lamprokostopoulou, George P. Chrousos, and Evangelia Charmandari. "Stress, the

Stress System and the Role of Glucocorticoids." *Neuroimmuno-modulation* 22, no. 1-2 (2015): 6-19.

11. Dhabhar, Firdaus S. "Enhancing versus Suppressive Effects of Stress on Immune Function: Implications for Immunoprotection and Immunopathology." *Neuroimmunomodulation* 16, no. 5 (2009): 300-317.

12. Cohen, S., D. Janicki-Deverts, W. J. Doyle, G. E. Miller, E. Frank, B. S. Rabin, and R. B. Turner. "Chronic Stress, Glucocorticoid Receptor Resistance, Inflammation, and Disease Risk." *Proceedings of the National Academy of Sciences* 109, no. 16 (2012): 5995-5999.

13. "Stressed in America." http://www.apa.org. http://www.apa.org/monitor/2011/01/stressed-america.aspx (accessed June 20, 2014).

Chapter 11

1. Centers for Disease Control and Prevention. "About BMI for Adults." http://www.cdc.gov/healthyweight/assessing/bmi/adult_bmi/index.html?s_cid=tw_ob064 (accessd July 11, 2014).

Acknowledgments

I could not have completed this book without the unwavering support of my husband, Justin, and our three beautiful daughters, Elly, Isla, and Ever. I love them endlessly. Their encouragement, curiosity, laughter and joy made every step of this project rewarding.

To my literary agent, Claire Gerus, who saw a glimmer of something special in this book long before it ever came to fruition.

To the entire team at Harlequin, especially my editor, Cara Bedick. Words cannot express my gratitude in how your talent and professionalism brought life to the pages of this book.

Index

About the Author

Traci D. Mitchell is one of America's leading weight loss experts. Taking a no-nonsense, relatable approach to motivating people to make positive changes in their life, Traci is a nationally recognized fitness, nutrition and weight loss professional who has been featured on *The Dr. Oz Show*, the *TODAY* show, *Steve Harvey*, as well as in *SELF* magazine, *SHAPE* magazine and on Oprah.com. A certified personal trainer and metabolic typing advisor, Traci has been helping people lose weight and get into great shape for over fifteen years. She holds a master's degree in communication from Marquette University and a master's in nutrition education from Hawthorn University. She lives in Chicago.

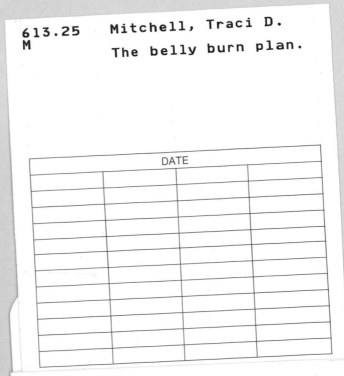

613.25   Mitchell, Traci D.
M   The belly burn plan.

DATE			